# Longevity
# Made Simple

# Longevity
## Made Simple

### HOW TO ADD

### 20 GOOD YEARS

### TO YOUR LIFE

Lessons from
Decades of Research

RICHARD J. FLANIGAN, MD

KATE FLANIGAN SAWYER, MD, MPH

Foreword by William Clifford Roberts, MD

WILLIAMS CLARK PUBLISHING, LLC

This book is intended as a reference volume only, not as a medical manual. It is sold with the understanding that neither the publisher nor the authors are rendering professional services. It is designed to provide accurate and authoritative information on its subject matter. The ideas, recommendations, and procedures contained herein are not intended as a substitute for any treatment that may have been prescribed by your physician or medical practitioner. The publisher and authors advise readers to take full responsibility for their well being and medical care. If you suspect you have a medical problem, we urge you to seek professional medical help.

Mention of companies, products, organizations, or authorities does not imply endorsements by the publisher or authors, nor does it imply that these companies, organizations, or authorities endorse the book, the authors, or the publisher.

Williams Clark books may be purchased for special sales, educational, business, or promotional uses. For more information, please write to: Special Markets Department, Williams Clark Publishing, LLC, 1218 Milwaukee St., Denver, CO 80206

Printed in the United States of America

First Edition

Book design by Jane Raese

Publisher's Cataloging-in-Publication Data
(Provided by Quality Books, Inc.)
Flanigan, Richard J.
Longevity made simple : how to add 20 good years to your life : lessons from decades of research / Richard J. Flanigan, Kate Flanigan Sawyer ; foreword by William C. Roberts.
p. cm.
Includes bibliographical references and index.
LCCN 2007926900
ISBN-13: 978-0-9792055-0-7
ISBN-10: 0-9792055-0-6
1. Longevity. 2. Health. I. Sawyer, Kate Flanigan. II. Title.
RA776.75.F53   2007   613
QBI07-600137

Distributed to the trade by Midpoint Trade Books.

Williams Clark Publishing, LLC
1218 Milwaukee St.
Denver, CO 80206

www.williamsclarkbooks.com

This book is joyously dedicated to Barbara, my fabulous wife.

*The stars were aligned 42 years ago with an improbable sighting*
*at a basketball game of a young lady who I would soon find out*
*I had so much in common with. She was:*
*a Flanigan (even spelled with an "i"),*
*a twin,*
*the youngest of 5 children.*
*You made this book happen with your enthusiastic encouragement.*
*Thank you, Barbara!*

—RICHARD J. FLANIGAN, MD

To my husband Mike, my biggest fan, my best friend.

—KATE FLANIGAN SAWYER, MD, MPH

# CONTENTS

# FOREWORD

For nearly three decades, I have collected more than 100 books on diet, nutrition, heart disease, and healthy living. Yet this splendid book by Dr. Richard Flanigan and his daughter, Dr. Kate Flanigan Sawyer, distinguishes itself with its brevity and unique approach. It does not limit itself to heart disease and nutrition, but focuses on the ten leading causes of death in the United States and what each of us can do—in cooperation with our physicians—to prevent them.

Surprisingly, a common thread is hidden beneath most of these health problems. Our lifestyle, not our genes, largely determines if and when we acquire one or more of the top ten diseases. Arterial disease (atherosclerosis, "blockages," "hardening of the arteries") is number one—our most common fatal or potentially fatal condition. The atherosclerotic gene is inherited by 1 in 500 individuals. The rest of us—499 of 500—determine whether we want plaques in our arteries and the major consequences of them, which include heart attacks, brain attacks (strokes) (number three), abdominal aortic aneurysm, and peripheral artery disease. Unfortunately, when we pull our chair up to the table twenty-one times every week, we eat the wrong calories and too many of them. As a consequence, our blood levels of cholesterol and glucose (sugar) rise, as do our blood pressure and waist measurements. All play major roles in heart disease, stroke, diabetes mellitus (number six) (most of those afflicted with diabetes die from heart attacks), kidney disease (number nine), and probably Alzheimer's disease (number eight).

It is the choices we make that usually trip us up. Drs. Flanigan and Sawyer help us make the right choices. They provide easy-to-follow guidelines and list twenty-two foods that are good for us and prevent plaque buildup.

Cancer (number two) has many things in common with heart disease. It's the food we eat that plays a major role in whether we get certain gastrointestinal cancers. For example, vegetarian-fruit eaters rarely get cancer of the colon, breast, or prostate gland, three of the four most common cancers. However, a strict vegetarian diet would eliminate fish and its superb benefits, including up to a 50 percent decrease in sudden death and 35 percent decrease in coronary artery disease and stroke. With that in mind, the authors advise eating several pure vegetarian meals each week and lots of fish—essentially a seafood/vegetarian diet, which is the diet I follow. When you do eat meat, the authors encourage you to limit your portions to the size of a deck of cards. They also advise eating slowly and leaving the table only 80 percent full.

And do not smoke! Smoking is responsible for 90 percent of all lung cancers, now far more common in women than breast cancer. Only 2 percent of physicians in the United States now smoke, compared to 21 percent of nonphysician adults. A pack of cigarettes (twenty cigarettes) in New York City now costs $8.00. If $8.00 were put into investments every day starting at age eighteen, all of us would be rich at sixty-five.

Remember to exercise for thirty minutes each day. It helps us maintain an ideal body weight and feel better all over—both mentally and physically. It also helps prevent all of the top ten fatal conditions.

The authors demonstrate the usefulness of many preventive drugs. Statins are to atherosclerosis what penicillin was to infectious disease. We have sixty-six antihypertensive drugs and twenty-seven combination drugs, so if your blood pressure is elevated, one, two, or possibly even three of these drugs should be taken every day. Hypertension plays a major role in stroke, which is exceedingly rare in people whose pressure is less than 120/80 mm Hg.

In summary, as Drs. Flanigan and Sawyer indicate, it's the choices we make that will most likely determine our fate. Those choices must be responsible ones. If you are overweight, it is good citizenship to lose weight. By doing so, your cholesterol levels fall, your blood pressure falls, your blood sugar falls, and, as a consequence, your arteries stay open and your organs receive their needed nutrition. Also, your risk for type 2 diabetes and chronic kidney disease drop precipitously.

With healthcare now utilizing 16 percent of our gross domestic product and with two-thirds of Americans overweight and half of them obese, each of us must do our share grabbing the wheel of health and steering down the healthy road. This book points us to that road.

I congratulate the authors for their wise counsel and urge all to follow it for a healthier, happier, and longer life.

*William Clifford Roberts, MD*
Executive Director
Baylor Heart and Vascular Institute
Editor-in-Chief, *The American Journal of Cardiology*

## PREFACE

This book can change your life. It is not a diet book, it is not an exercise book, it is a *longevity* book: a book that explains in simple language what science tells us about living long, healthy lives.

Only 3 percent of the population practices the four standard healthy habits: they do not smoke, they follow a nutritious diet, they exercise regularly, and they keep their weight under control. It is staggering to imagine that 97 percent of the U.S. population does not do these four things. And even our health professionals' habits are abysmal. Only 4 percent of almost forty-three thousand health professionals in the Harvard-based Health Professionals Follow-Up Study adhered to the above four healthy habits, plus a fifth healthy habit—consuming one to two alcoholic beverages per day.

Clearly, there is a dire need for action and reliable information about healthy habits that can prevent disease.

Our interest in prevention dates back to about 1977 when high-density lipoprotein (HDL) was discovered. Research showed that this cholesterol was actually good for you and that increased HDL levels can significantly reduce deaths due to heart disease.

As authors, clinicians, and prevention specialists, we spend an enormous amount of time scouring the research literature to find and to present important new information about prevention. For many years, I, Richard J. Flanigan, have been a member of a prevention journal club here in Denver. Our mission is to present data that make a difference, that will inform our practice habits, and that will improve and lengthen our patients' lives. We review thirty-nine journals and newsletters monthly.

Through our research and experience, we have learned what our patients can do to add good years to their lives and to lower their risks of dying from heart disease, stroke, and cancer. We now get the chance to share with you, the reader, our investigation and analysis of the evidence-based data.

Our objective is to bring simplicity and clarity to powerful but often bewildering, and sometimes contradictory, medical and health information. In *Longevity Made Simple*, we have worked hard to provide you with simple guidelines to increase your lifespan.

We hope you enjoy this book. Better yet, we hope you learn from it.

*Richard J. Flanigan, MD*
*Kate Flanigan Sawyer, MD, MPH*

## ACKNOWLEDGMENTS

What a joy to thank the many people who have offered me encouragement and direction while writing this book. I'd especially like to thank my co-author and daughter, Kate. Since Kate was in pigtails, we have shared a passion for health and fitness, and a love of knowledge.

My wife, Barbara; my children and their spouses, Conn (Monica), Kate (Mike), Regan, and Dan (Erin); and my grandchildren, Delaney, Bryn, Eleri, Ryan, Kathleen, and Sienna, have tirelessly cheered me on in my athletic and professional endeavors. I am deeply grateful to every one of you (and to my seventh grandchild who is due to arrive soon!). You have given me your unconditional love and support and occasional doses of humorous ribbing!

My identical twin brother, Don, a radiologist and rower, has helped me appreciate the value of pursuing my goals, win or lose, and of living life to its fullest. I have also had the unwavering support of my other siblings, Father Ted Flanigan, Sister Regina Flanigan, and Dr. Eleanor Flanigan, as well as many nephews and nieces. Thanks also to Dianne Flanigan  and John Elias, our wonderful in-laws.

To my patients I owe humble thanks. I am honored to share in your lives and inspired by your dedication to healthy living.

In my practice, I am fortunate to be surrounded by a highly capable staff. Special kudos go to Mari Baerren, who started as my secretary thirty-three years ago and is now a trustworthy and devoted office manager. I'd also like to thank Lori Kosty, my nurse; Kathy Roberts, echo technician; and Marsha Witzman, receptionist.

A warm thank you goes to Arthur Agatston, MD, whose book *The South Beach Diet* is still the best we have.

Thanks to the Denver Prevention Journal Club and its members Wayne Peters, MD, James Ehrlich, MD, Jack Locke, MD, Robert Eckel, MD, and John Hokenson, PhD. Meeting with this group has been enormously stimulating and enlightening.

I owe a special thanks to Richard Collins, MD, "The Cooking Cardiologist," and Brenda Lambert, RN, MBA, for allowing us to use the delicious and "simple" recipes from Dr. Collins's excellent book *Cooking with Heart.*

I want to single out four of my medical heroes for their influence and inspiration: William Clifford Roberts, MD, for his enthusiastic support and for instilling in me a passion to fight atherosclerosis; Gilbert S. Blount, MD, for stellar cardiology training; William Castelli, MD, for increasing my love for cardiovascular prevention; and Kenneth Cooper, MD, for fervor of the exercise component in prevention.

I have several sports heroes who made a huge impact on me, including Allen Rosenberg (1964 gold-medal-winning Olympic coach for eight-oared shell), who was an outstanding leader and mentor. The late John B. Kelly of Philadelphia instilled a gracious competitiveness in me and the rest of his rowers at Vesper Boat Club. The late Tibor Machan, a renowned rowing coach from Hungary, came to the Vesper Boat Club and made it world class; I appreciate his faith in my brother Don and me.

I owe a debt of gratitude to Nancy Peterson, Doug Stackhouse, Sharon Martin, Adelaide Fletcher, Pam Roth, Dorothy Struble, and the late Mary DeMund of the Denver Medical Library staff. They are the most competent librarians imaginable.

Last, but surely not least, both Kate and I want to thank Kathleen Kauff and William Allstetter of Williams Clark Publishing, our publisher and friends, who believed in our passion and worked so hard to make our message come to life.

*Richard J. Flanigan, MD*

Gratefully I thank my family, friends, and teachers, who have provided the guidance and support to encourage me to write on my favorite subject, longevity.

Thanks to the 9HealthFair, particularly Angie Devlin and Jim Goddard, for providing an opportunity and outlet to promote our mutual perspective on healthy living and disease prevention.

I want to acknowledge my family—all the Sawyers and Flanigans—who have demonstrated unending love and support not only for the book, but also for my career, for my well being, and for my husband and children. In particular, I want to thank my sister Regan for her patience, her constant friendship, and help with all areas of my life. And I want to thank my mom, who has helped me become the person that I am, guided me through many of life's challenges, and always reminded me to put things into perspective.

Thanks to my husband, Mike. We went through it all together: grueling years of medical school, residencies, and internships; moving across country and back; having a family; writing a book—no one else in the world could have made such demanding, sleep-deprived years so much fun. Looking back, it didn't seem so hard after all! And to Ryan and Kathleen—I am so blessed to have two children as wonderful as you.

Finally, without my dad, there would be no book. Since I was a very young child, my dad and I bonded over a mutual passion for prevention. His enthusiasm for health promotion and disease prevention rubbed off on me and has helped me find and construct what I would consider to be the perfect career. Thanks, Dad. I'm proud to be a chip off the old block!

*Kate Flanigan Sawyer, MD, MPH*

# Longevity
# Made Simple

## CHAPTER 1

# A Great Time to Live a Long Life

How long do you want to live? If you are reading this book, you probably want to live as long and healthy a life as possible. Well, you are in luck. Today, we live in a unique time in human history. People are living longer than they ever have before.

Back when Julius Caesar ruled the Roman Empire, in the first century B.C., the average human life span was twenty-two years. That's a pretty grim number. Imagine living only twenty-two years! However, during the next two thousand years, the average life span slowly crept up. By 1900 the average human could expect to live to the ripe old age of forty-seven.

The main causes of death between Caesar's time and the early nineteen hundreds were infections. For example, if you look at the leading causes of death in 1860, eight of the top ten killers were infectious diseases: tuberculosis, diarrhea, cholera, pneumonia, diphtheria, dysentery, scarlet fever, and nephritis. Infantile convulsions and infantile stroke were the only noninfectious diseases among the

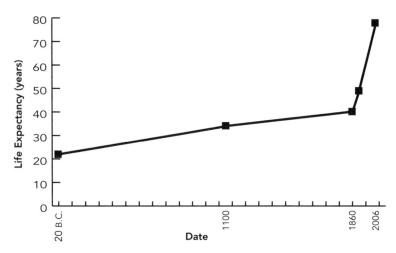

**Life Expectancy Since Julius Caesar**

*Sources:* U.S. Centers for Disease Control and Prevention; Lydia Bronte, *The Longevity Factor,* HarperCollins Publishers, 1993; Human Mortality Database, University of California, Berkeley (USA), and Max Planck Institute for Demographic Research (Germany).

top ten killers, accounting for 9 percent of deaths. So, for nearly two thousand years, 91 percent of the population died of infections.

Then, in 1928, a Scottish scientist named Alexander Fleming discovered penicillin. This groundbreaking discovery ushered in the age of antibiotics, which changed everything. Bacterial infections were essentially eliminated as a major cause of death, and today they no longer have a significant effect on the longevity of our population. Rather than losing 91 percent of our population to infections, only 3 to 4 percent of people in the developed world die from bacterial infections.

That, in turn, has dramatically increased our longevity. Between 1900 and 2000, the average life span in the United States jumped thirty years, from forty-seven to almost seventy-eight. We have never lived longer. Why, then, write a book on longevity? Because we can tell you how to live even longer *and* better.

## DO YOU WANT TO LIVE TO 100?

The average life span for a person born in America today is seventy-eight years. This number may sound good, but it's only an average, which means that many people do not make it to this age. When you take a closer look at the current statistics, the news is, indeed, more sobering. One-third of the American public dies before age sixty-five. Only half of us make it to the age of seventy-eight. In addition, many people who do live this long are ill, suffering, or disabled by chronic disease.

When we ask our patients if they want to live to 100, most of them say, "No way!" They say this because they envision their final years as dreadful ones dominated by illness, disability, and frailty. What our patients tell us they do want is quality. They want to remain healthy and active for as long as possible.

It just so happens that what gives us quality also gives us quantity. So, in our quest for greater longevity, we can also expect to enjoy better quality of life. Maybe living to 100 wouldn't be so bad after all.

## LIFE WITHOUT DISEASE: UTOPIA OR REALITY?

Have you ever wondered how long you could live if you had a life without disease? Well, Dr. William Schwartz, a professor of internal medicine at the University of Southern California who studies the human genome, addressed that question in his book *Life without Disease: The Pursuit of Medical Utopia.* Dr. Schwartz believes that scientists are going to find the longevity gene in our lifetime. Once that is achieved, he also believes we will be able to double our life span and live nearly 150 years. While we are not so sure that scientists will discover a longevity gene anytime soon, there is ample evidence that we already have the tools to live longer, healthier lives.

## The Real Number-One Killer—Artery Disease

In this book, we treat heart disease and stroke as different diseases, in part because the U.S. Centers for Disease Control and Prevention classify them as independent causes of death. But, in reality, they are similar diseases; they both result from problems in the arteries that disrupt the supply of oxygenated blood to your heart and brain. (See "It's really about the arteries" on page 12, to learn how arteries become blocked.)

So, in essence, heart disease and stroke are really artery diseases. Physicians group all problems of blood supply under a single name: cardiovascular disease. Cardiovascular disease includes not only stroke and coronary artery disease, but also high blood pressure, heart failure, and a few other circulatory diseases as well.

Artery disease, or bad blood supply, is the real number-one killer in America. According to the American Heart Association, cardiovascular disease was the underlying cause in 37.3 percent of all deaths in 2003, or one in 2.7 deaths. More alarming, cardiovascular disease was a contributing cause of death in 58 percent of all deaths.

As the famed nutrition and cholesterol expert Scott Grundy, MD, PhD, once wrote—"you are as old as your arteries." If your arteries are stiff and clogged with cholesterol, then you are not likely to live long. On the other hand, if your arteries are resilient and free of cholesterol plaques, you are likely to enjoy many more years of life no matter how many years you have already lived on this planet. So, remember, if you want to live a long life, treat your arteries well.

Dr. Thomas Perls, a researcher at Boston University, is the head of the New England Centenarian Study. He has extensively interviewed people who lived to 100 in order to understand the factors that contribute to longevity. Dr. Perls believes that we are genetically capable of living to at least eighty-five, but that lifestyle choices we make can alter this number drastically in either direction. We wholeheartedly agree with Dr. Perls. And that is the crux of this book. We believe that choices you make today about your lifestyle, about the medications you take, and about the screening tests you get can extend your life twenty to twenty-five years, or even more.

Why do we think this? First, let us remember what has happened during the past century. With the advent of antibiotics and the widespread use of vaccines, infectious diseases have almost been eliminated as major killers in the developed world. (Infectious diseases do remain a leading cause of death in the developing world, however, because of poor sanitation and limited access to medications.) As a result, the average life span has increased by thirty years, or more than 60 percent.

So, if you want to add another twenty to thirty years to your life, you need to understand, treat, and prevent the diseases that cause most of the deaths today. What kills most people in the developed world today? Read on.

## TOP TEN CAUSES OF DEATH

*Death is not popular, it is not good for the complexion,*
*and it leaves you with too much time on your hands.*
—GEORGE BURNS, 1896–1996

Do you have any idea how many diseases there are? In our office we have a big, thick book called the *International Statistical Classification of Diseases and Related Health Problems,* Tenth Revision, or *ICD-10*, which is a catalog of known diseases. When we see patients, we have to code their disorders using this book. It contains codes for more than 100,000 diseases. However, nearly 60 percent of the U.S. population dies from just three causes: heart disease, cancer, and stroke.

## Top Ten Causes of Death in the United States, 2003

| Rank | Cause | Percentage of Deaths | Number of Deaths |
|------|-------|---------------------|------------------|
| 1 | Heart disease | 28 | 685,000 |
| 2 | Cancer | 23 | 557,000 |
| 3 | Stroke | 6 | 158,000 |
| 4 | Chronic obstructive pulmonary disease (COPD) | 5 | 126,000 |
| 5 | Accidents | 4 | 109,000 |
| 6 | Diabetes mellitus | 3 | 74,000 |
| 7 | Influenza/pneumonia | 3 | 65,000 |
| 8 | Alzheimer's disease | 3 | 63,000 |
| 9 | Kidney disease | 2 | 42,000 |
| 10 | Septicemia | 1 | 34,000 |
| | **Total of all 10 causes** | 78 | 1,913,000 |

*Source:* U.S. Centers for Disease Control and Prevention, "National Vital Statistics Reports," 54, no. 13 (April 19, 2006).

Twenty-eight percent of us die from heart disease. Twenty-three percent die from cancer. Stroke accounts for another 6 percent of deaths in the United States.

The fourth leading cause of death is chronic obstructive pulmonary disease, almost always due to smoking tobacco, which kills 5 percent of us. Four percent will die from accidents, and 3 percent will die from complications due to diabetes mellitus. That number, however, downplays the significance of diabetes because 65 to 75 percent of diabetics die from a vascular problem such as heart disease or stroke. Three percent die from the infectious diseases flu and pneumonia. Another 3 percent die from Alzheimer's disease, and 2 percent from kidney disease. Rounding out the top ten causes of death in America is septicemia, which is the clinical name for blood poisoning, an infection that kills 1 percent of us.

The top ten causes account for almost 80 percent of all deaths in the United States. And not one of the diseases beyond the top ten accounts for even 1 percent of deaths. So, to live a long and healthy life, the odds suggest we needn't worry much about the vast majority of 100,000 diseases listed in the *ICD-10*. Instead, we should focus on preventing and treating just ten of them.

## WHAT DETERMINES LONGEVITY?

Can we find a modern-day cure, comparable to antibiotics, for today's top ten killers? Many people think not. They believe that their time on this earth is predestined by two immutable factors: family history and genetics.

We disagree. Family history and genetics do play a role in your longevity, but not as much as most people think. Lifestyle choices you make—diet, exercise, medications, and screening tests—can reduce the impact of those factors and greatly increase your longevity. The INTERHEART study, involving 29,000 patients from 52 countries, pointed out that lifestyle risk factors predict 90–94 percent of all heart disease. Genetics, therefore, contributes 10 percent or less of your risk of heart disease.

Many people believe that if you have cancer in your family history and in your genes, there is nothing you can do about it. But careful study has shown that much of the time this is not the case. In 1981 a landmark study published in the *Journal of the National Cancer Institute* concluded that diet plays a role in most cancers, contributing to as much as 90 percent of all stomach and colon cancer cases. Tobacco accounts for more than 90 percent of all lung cancers. So it is largely the choices that you make—your diet and tobacco use— that help determine whether you get cancer.

This is not to say that family history and genetics play no role in cancer, or that cancer does not sometimes seem to strike at random. We can't completely control the diseases we get, but we can dramatically alter the odds in our favor. And it is not only cancer and heart disease we're talking about. As we will discuss later in this book, the chances that you will suffer a stroke, develop diabetes, or die of any of the other leading causes of death can be dramatically altered by choices you make about diet, exercise, medication, and medical screening.

## YOU CHOOSE

That is why we wrote this book: to help you make the choices that will help you live a long and healthy life. What are those choices? And how do you make them? Fortunately, over the past thirty to forty years, thousands of researchers in the United States and around the world have been studying which diseases kill us, what causes them, and how to prevent them.

We have studied that research—not just the report that was published last week or last month, but also studies from the past decades that have withstood the test of time, sound and consistent research that is based on lengthy clinical trials involving thousands of people. We have also learned from our patients what they have done to improve their lives and to lower their risks of dying from the most common deadly diseases.

Based on what we have learned, we have come up with simple, effective, research-based guidelines to increase the length and quality of your life.

## YOUR RISK PROFILE

We have already identified the top ten killers in America today. In Chapter 2 we tell you more about those killers and the risk factors that most commonly contribute to them, including high blood pressure, high cholesterol, and lack of exercise. In Chapter 3 we help you develop your own personal risk profile, the combination of risk factors that most threaten your health and longevity. Your risk profile will help you develop your own unique longevity plan, one that addresses your most important risk factors and is most likely to increase your life span. Chapters 4 through 9 outline simple, effective steps you can take to control those risk factors.

So, after identifying and reducing your personal risks, the next best thing you can do to prevent disease is to detect it before it spreads. In Chapter 10 we recommend a host of screening tests that will help you not only identify and monitor risk factors but also detect the earliest signs of disease so that you can take action to treat it or to prevent its progression. In Chapter 11, we will put it all together with ten essential tips that can add twenty quality years to your life.

## TAKE RESPONSIBILITY

The next step is yours. We can provide you with information and guidance. But, in the end, your health is up to you. You decide what you put in your mouth, what you do with your body, or what screening tests you get. What we are telling you here is that those choices make a real difference. The right choices can add years to your life, while the wrong ones can not only take away years, but also make those final years low quality ones filled with disease and disability.

So, we urge you to be aggressive about your health. Learn your personal risk factors, take the necessary steps to control them, and make plans for a longer, healthier, and happier life.

## CHAPTER 2

# Understanding the Biggest Threats to Your Longevity

As we outlined in the first chapter, the ten leading causes of death in the United States account for almost 80 percent of all deaths. The top three diseases alone account for 57 percent of deaths. So, if you can understand and prevent the ten most deadly diseases, you can dramatically improve your chances of living a longer and healthier life.

In this chapter we briefly describe the ten most deadly diseases, what causes them, and the risk factors that increase your chances of developing them.

## NO. 1 KILLER: HEART DISEASE— STARTS EARLY, BUT REVERSIBLE

There's an old "Peanuts" comic strip that shows Snoopy jogging. Snoopy's feet are complaining, his knees are throbbing, his back is aching, and he has a stitch in his side. Meanwhile, his brain exclaims to the other parts of the body, "Have you ever thought about why we're doing this? Just to keep the heart in shape!"

In the next panel, Snoopy's heart replies, "Just remember, boys, if I go, you all go."

We can't emphasize enough how true this statement really is. You can have sore ankles, a bad back, a skin rash, and a headache, but none of these ailments will kill you. Ultimately, to stay alive, you are dependent on your heart to circulate oxygenated blood to the rest of your body and organs. Quite simply, you require a functioning, healthy heart to live.

The heart is an amazing muscle. It beats more than 100,000 times a day, every day, without ever stopping to rest, for more than seventy-five years on average. It won't let you down . . . unless you let it down with bad habits, poor diet, and lack of regular exercise.

Regrettably, Americans are letting their hearts down in a big way, leading to an epidemic of heart disease in our country. Heart disease is the leading cause of death in the United States, accounting for more than 650,000 deaths each year. The vast majority of these deaths are caused by heart attacks due to atherosclerosis.

### It's really about the arteries

Diseased coronary arteries are the underlying cause of the dreaded and often deadly heart attack. Arteries can become diseased with atherosclerosis, which chokes off blood flow and thereby deprives your heart muscles of vital oxygen.

When heart-muscle cells are deprived of oxygen, they begin to die. That is a heart attack. The size of the heart attack depends upon the size of the artery that is blocked; the larger the blocked artery, the more muscle tissue is deprived of oxygen and the larger the heart at-

## Lori's Story: Reversal of Atherosclerosis

Lori, my nurse, is 37 years old. Before beginning statin medications she had disturbingly high cholesterol levels, as high as 407 mg/dL. She began taking a statin in 1992. As of March 2006 her cholesterol had dropped to about 250 mg/dL. We wanted to get it even lower.

First, we did two baseline vascular studies to evaluate the state of her arteries. The arterial elasticity test, which measures how supple or elastic the arteries are, showed that her arteries were abnormally stiff. The other test was a carotid ultrasound with carotid intima-media thickness (CIMT). The carotid ultrasound showed a small plaque in the right carotid and plaque in about 5 to 10 percent of the left carotid. Both arteries had thick CIMTs of 0.9mm. We doubled her statin medication.

Six months later we repeated these vascular studies. Her arterial elasticity had changed from abnormal to normal. The plaque in the right carotid had completely disappeared, and the plaque in the left carotid was one-third its original size. The CIMT had also reverted back to normal, 0.6 mm, on the right and 0.4 mm on the left.

This wonderful story corroborates what we know about reversal—that it can occur and quite rapidly. *–Richard J. Flanigan, MD*

tack. Each year more than a million people in the United States have a heart attack, and about half of them die.

Atherosclerosis is a term that comes from Greek: "athero" for fat and "sclerosis" for hardening. So, in essence, the word means "hardening of the arteries due to fat deposits." But the fat deposits of atherosclerosis are actually a complicated mix of cholesterol, inflammatory cells, scar tissue, and calcium.

Take a look at the picture of an artery timeline on page 14. This picture describes the process of developing atherosclerosis, or coronary artery disease.

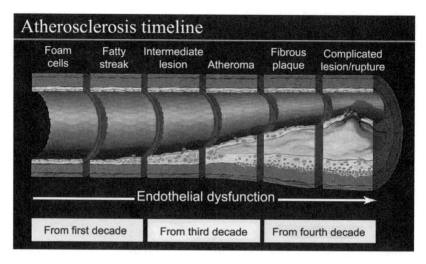

## Atherosclerosis timeline

| Foam cells | Fatty streak | Intermediate lesion | Atheroma | Fibrous plaque | Complicated lesion/rupture |

Endothelial dysfunction →

| From first decade | From third decade | From fourth decade |

*Atherosclerosis can trigger heart attacks and strokes when plaques rupture.* (*Source:* Adapted from Carl J. Pepine, "The effects of angiotensin-converting enzyme inhibition on endothelial dysfunction: potential role in myocardial ischemia," *The American Journal of Cardiology* 82 [August 6, 1998], 23S-27S.)

Atherosclerosis begins with an injury to the blood vessel's inner-most layer of cells, called the endothelium. The damage can be caused by high blood pressure or something in your blood stream, such as tobacco toxins, inflammation, or even blood sugar.

Once the endothelium is damaged, LDL cholesterol (the "bad" cholesterol—see page 36) enters the artery wall and begins accumulating.

At the same time, the immune system attempts to repair the damage by recruiting cells to the site of the injury. This inflammatory process is the same one that occurs when your scraped knee becomes red and swollen. The problem is that this inflammatory response actually contributes to the damage by adding to the size of the plaque and creating scar tissue. Now there is a big gob of LDL cholesterol, immune-system cells, and scar tissue, which is called a plaque, growing inside your artery wall. If it grows big enough, plaque can block the blood vessel and starve the muscles downstream of vital oxygen.

The size of the plaque is important, but recent research shows that the stability of the plaque is just as important, if not more so. An unstable plaque can rupture and cause a clot, even if the artery is only 50 percent blocked. In fact, one important study found that the majority of heart attacks are caused by plaques that block less than half of the artery. The process of damaging an artery, therefore, is not just about the cholesterol plaque. It is actually an interplay of three main factors: plaque, inflammation, and clotting. And the problem is that once the process has started, it is likely to continue—unless something is done to stop the progression of the disease, such as taking medication or modifying risk factors.

Most strokes are also caused by atherosclerosis, which leads to the blockage of blood vessels in the brain and the death of brain cells.

Now you know how important it is to prevent the atherosclerotic process from starting and to keep your arteries healthy. Healthy arteries are the key to keeping your organs alive.

### Developing heart disease: The good news and the bad news

We always like to start with the good news, which is that heart disease takes decades to develop and is preventable, even reversible. Many early animal studies show that while atherosclerosis (deposition of fat in the arteries) can easily be induced by a high-fat, high-cholesterol diet, it can also be *reversed* by a healthy diet.

Research continues to demonstrate that this reversal of atherosclerosis can occur in humans as well. The Asteroid Trial, of 349 patients on cholesterol-lowering medications for two years, showed "bad" LDL levels cut in half, "good" HDL levels boosted by almost 15 percent, and fatty deposits inside arteries, known as plaques, reduced by 7 percent.

A review of nine different studies also showed a significant reduction in plaque volume when people lowered their LDL levels to below 100 mg/dL. (For an explanation of the different forms of cholesterol, see page 36.)

Now the bad news: the first signs of heart disease develop as early as the first decade of life. Researchers looked at the arteries of American soldiers who fought in the Korean War and died on the battlefield. In 1953, these researchers reported that more than three-quarters of the GIs, whose average age was twenty-two, had visible evidence of coronary atherosclerosis. Additionally, autopsies of children who died from accidents or suicides showed that the disease process leading to atherosclerosis has often begun in children as young as ten years old.

Hence, research suggests that it's never too early to teach, encourage, and practice preventive lifestyle behaviors, such as getting regular physical activity, eating a healthy diet, and not using tobacco products. Your lifestyle choices can prevent atherosclerosis from even starting.

| Major Risk Factors for Heart Disease |
| :--- |
| ▶ Elevated cholesterol |
| ▶ High blood pressure |
| ▶ Lack of regular exercise |
| ▶ Poor diet |
| ▶ Tobacco use |
| ▶ Diabetes |
| ▶ Family history |
| ▶ Age |
| ▶ Gender |

## NO. 2 KILLER: CANCER— MORE PREVENTABLE THAN YOU THINK

Cancer is the second biggest cause of death in America. Everyone we know has been touched by this disease, whether they're battling cancer themselves or a family member or close friend has been diag-

## What Is Cancer?

Cancer develops when damage to your DNA causes cells in your body to divide and multiply uncontrollably. In normal conditions, your body is able to repair damage to DNA. In cancer cells, damaged DNA is not repaired. We can inherit damaged DNA, which accounts for the genetics of cancer. More often, however, one's DNA becomes damaged by exposure to something harmful, such as tobacco smoke.

nosed with it. The lifetime probability of developing cancer is 46 percent for men and 38 percent for women. The risk of dying of cancer is one in four for men and one in five for women.

It's a scary word—cancer. Many people believe that cancer is something that strikes randomly, like lightning—almost as if you were in the wrong place at the wrong time. Others believe it will never happen to them. We recently had a patient who claimed he would never get cancer, even though he had been smoking two packs of cigarettes a day for thirty years. "My parents both lived into their eighties, and they smoked like chimneys," he stated. "Cancer just doesn't happen in my family."

That is not an accurate view of cancer. Genetic inheritance does influence your risk for cancer. However, lifestyle and environmental factors play an even larger role.

In the late 1970s, the U.S. Congress commissioned two British epidemiologists, Richard Doll and Richard Peto, to estimate the extent to which cancer is avoidable. Their landmark study, published in the *Journal of the National Cancer Institute* in 1981, concluded that tobacco and diet were the major cancer-causing culprits. Workplace pollutants accounted for a relatively minor 4 percent of cancer cases.

This seminal work further developed our knowledge of the relationship among food, nutrition, and cancer. Doll and Peto agreed with previous research that found overconsumption of fat and meat to be major contributors to cancer. They also noted the preventive effects of fiber and of dietary antioxidants in fruits and vegetables.

Doll and Peto estimated that dietary changes could reduce U.S. cancer death rates by up to 90 percent for stomach and large bowel cancers; 50 percent for breast, uterus, gallbladder, and pancreatic cancers; 20 percent for larynx, bladder, cervix, mouth, pharynx, and esophagus cancers; and 10 percent for other cancers.

> ## Major Risk Factors for Cancer
>
> ▶ Tobacco use
> ▶ Excess weight
> ▶ Lack of regular physical activity
> ▶ Inadequate consumption of fruits and vegetables
> ▶ Overconsumption of fats
> ▶ Overconsumption of processed and red meats
> ▶ Intake of more than two alcoholic beverages a day for men, one for women
> ▶ Family history
> ▶ Age

More recently, the 2006 "American Cancer Society Guidelines on Nutrition and Physical Activity for Cancer Prevention" offers a wealth of evidence and suggestions about lifestyle changes people can make to reduce the chances of developing cancer, such as exercise, eating more fruits and vegetables, and using sunscreen.

So, just because your grandmother or uncle died of cancer does not necessarily mean you will get cancer. By reading this book, you will better understand your risks and, if necessary, learn how to modify your behavior to greatly reduce your own chances of developing cancer.

## NO. 3 KILLER: STROKE—
## A DEVASTATING "BRAIN ATTACK"

A stroke is devastating. If a stroke doesn't kill you, it is likely to leave you permanently disabled and dependent on others for your care. Stroke is the third leading cause of death and a leading cause of long-term disability in America today.

The majority of strokes, about 83 percent, are what we call ischemic strokes. An ischemic stroke is essentially a "brain attack." A blood vessel supplying oxygenated blood to part of the brain is blocked, just as a coronary artery is blocked in a heart attack. Starved of oxygen, the brain cells die. The size and location of the artery that is blocked determines the extent and severity of the stroke.

Blockages are caused by three things: (1) a clot in the artery supplying blood to the brain; (2) a piece of a clot forms elsewhere, breaks off, travels to the brain, and blocks an artery there; or (3) a severe narrowing of an artery caused solely by atherosclerosis. Ischemic strokes are preventable, in the same way that ischemic heart disease is preventable.

The other common type of stroke is hemorrhagic, which accounts for 17 percent of all strokes.

### Major Risk Factors for Stroke

- High blood pressure
- High cholesterol
- Tobacco use
- Lack of physical exercise
- Poor diet
- Diabetes

### Secondary Risk Factors

- Age—risk doubles for each decade over age fifty-five
- Family history of stroke
- Birth control pills
- Atrial fibrillation
- Heart failure
- Excess alcohol
- Prior stroke or heart attack
- Carotid artery disease
- African descent
- Female gender

## Know the Symptoms of a Stroke

The American Heart Association recently conducted a telephone survey of more than one thousand women over twenty-five years of age. They found that only one out of three women correctly identified the warning signs of stroke. This is worrisome because early treatment can greatly reduce the risk of permanent disability and death.

Your or a loved one's life could depend on knowing the warning signals. If you are experiencing or see any of the signs below, call 911 immediately.

**Warning signs of stroke:**

▸ Sudden numbness or weakness in the face, arm, or leg (especially on one side of the body)
▸ Sudden confusion, trouble speaking or understanding
▸ Sudden problems seeing in one eye or both eyes
▸ Sudden dizziness, loss of balance or coordination, or trouble walking
▸ Sudden severe headaches with no known cause

*Source:* American Stroke Association, http://www.strokeassociation.org.

Hemorrhagic strokes occur when a blood vessel in the brain weakens and ruptures. The ruptures occur as a result of high blood pressure or weakened vessel walls. Blood leaks into the brain instead of continuing on its path to nourish brain cells farther down the circulatory system. The effect of hemorrhagic strokes is the same as that for ischemic strokes: brain cells are deprived of oxygen and die.

## NO. 4 KILLER: CHRONIC OBSTRUCTIVE PULMONARY DISEASE (COPD)—ALSO CAUSED BY TOBACCO

People always associate smoking with lung cancer. But smoking tobacco causes almost as many cases of chronic obstructive pulmonary disease (COPD) as it does lung cancer. COPD is the fourth leading cause of death in the United States. A full 90 percent of the cases are caused by smoking tobacco.

Chronic obstructive pulmonary disease is a term that refers to two lung diseases, chronic bronchitis and emphysema. Often these conditions occur together. Chronic bronchitis results from inflammation and eventual scarring of the bronchial tubes, which leads to a mucus-producing cough and infections in the airways, both of which make it difficult to breathe. Emphysema refers to the gradual and permanent destruction of tiny air sacs in the lungs, known as alveoli. As these air sacs are destroyed, the lungs transfer less oxygen to the bloodstream, resulting in a shortness of breath that is particularly noticeable when exhaling.

Unfortunately, there is no cure for COPD. But you can prevent it by not smoking or by quitting before you develop it. And even if you

### Major Risk Factors for COPD

▸ Smoking tobacco accounts for 90 percent of cases of COPD.
▸ Genetics—There is an inherited form of COPD, known as alpha-1 antitrypsin disease, responsible for 5 percent (at most) of the cases.
▸ The other 5 percent of cases may be attributed to air pollution, second-hand smoke, history of childhood respiratory infections, and occupational exposure to certain industrial pollutants.

have been diagnosed with COPD, quitting can help slow the progression of the disease and delay death.

## NO. 5 KILLER: ACCIDENTS—
## NOT JUST A THREAT TO THE YOUNG

Unintentional injuries, the fifth leading cause of death, kill about 110,000 people in the United States every year. Motor vehicle accidents are the single biggest cause of accidental death, accounting for forty-five thousand deaths each year. Accidental poisonings kill about twenty thousand people, and unintentional falls kill seventeen thousand people.

We tend to think of accidental deaths occurring only to young people. Indeed, they are relatively high in the first year of life, with drown-

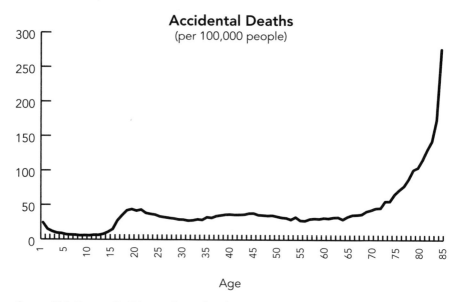

**Accidental Deaths**
(per 100,000 people)

*Source:* U.S. Centers for Disease Control and Prevention, "National Vital Statistics Reports," 52, no. 21 (June 2, 2004), Table 11.

ing and suffocation causing the most deaths among infants. However, the number of accidental deaths are low between ages one and fourteen. They begin rising again at age fifteen and peak at twenty-one. Motor vehicle accidents cause the most deaths in the fifteen-to-thirty-year-old range, peaking at age twenty-five, and dropping thereafter.

All forms of accidental death begin rising sharply at age sixty-five, and by age seventy-five are higher than at any other time in our lives. At age seventy-five and beyond, falls become a major cause of accidental death, as do motor vehicle accidents and suffocation. For women, deaths from falls increase fivefold between the ages of sixty-five and eighty-five.

So buckle up, exercise, eat well, accident-proof your home for both the young and the old, and, whatever you do, don't drink and drive!

### Risk Factors for Accidents

▶ Age
▶ Alcohol/drugs
▶ Lack of exercise/coordination
▶ Vision or hearing impairment, physical disabilities
▶ Lack of seat belt use
▶ Icy, slippery conditions
▶ Fatigue
▶ Poor lighting
▶ Certain medications
▶ Lack of child-safety practices: locks, window openings, hot water

## NO. 6 KILLER: DIABETES— ATTACK ON EVERY PART OF YOUR BODY

Talk about diseases you don't want to get! There are not many chronic diseases out there that can cause as much damage to your entire body as uncontrolled diabetes. Diabetes adversely affects your

## Adverse Effects of Diabetes on Your Body

- ▶ Heart disease and stroke—kill 65–75 percent of diabetics
- ▶ High blood pressure—found in 73 percent of diabetics
- ▶ Kidney disease and failure, leading to dialysis
- ▶ Eye problems leading to blindness
- ▶ Nerve damage and neuropathy
- ▶ Foot complications and amputations
- ▶ Skin complications—infections and poor wound healing
- ▶ Depression
- ▶ Complications in pregnancy—birth defects, stillbirths, and large babies
- ▶ Sexual dysfunction
- ▶ Dental disease

eyes, kidneys, nerves, toes, blood vessels, heart, and brain. It also hampers your ability to heal after a wound.

There are two types of diabetes: 1 and 2. Both are related to problems with the hormone insulin. Insulin tells our cells to absorb sugar, in the form of glucose, and convert it into the energy required for living. When there is no insulin or when cells don't get its message, glucose continues circulating in your bloodstream, which is not good. Glucose is a large molecule that often binds with hemoglobin or LDL cholesterol in your blood. This large complex can get stuck in tight places, such as vessels in your eyes, leading to blindness, or vessels in your kidneys, leading to kidney failure. Recently, scientists have come to appreciate that glucose can also damage the endothelium (the blood vessel's innermost layer of cells) in medium and large arteries, leading to atherosclerosis. As a result, 65 percent of diabetics die of stroke or heart disease, while only 4 percent die of complications from diabetes itself.

In type 1 diabetes, also known as juvenile diabetes, the body does not produce insulin. It must be supplied through injections. Type 1 diabetes is primarily a genetic disease.

Type 2 diabetes, the most common type of diabetes, is related to obesity and poor lifestyle choices. In type 2 diabetes, either the body does not produce enough insulin or cells in the body don't respond well to the insulin that is produced.

Unfortunately, type 2 diabetes is becoming increasingly prevalent. More than twenty million people in the United States have diabetes. An additional forty-one million people have a condition referred to as "pre-diabetes," in which blood glucose levels are higher than normal, but not all the way to diabetic levels.

## Major Risk Factors for Type 2 Diabetes

▸ Being overweight or obese
▸ Family history
▸ Lack of physical exercise
▸ High blood pressure
▸ Low HDL cholesterol
▸ High triglycerides
▸ History of vascular disease
▸ History of gestational diabetes
▸ Delivery of a baby weighing over nine pounds
▸ Being of African, Hispanic, Native American, Asian, or Pacific Islander descent
▸ Being over age forty-five

We now know that even pre-diabetes affects your health adversely. In fact, in the June 2006 issue of the medical journal *Diabetes Care,* researchers found that pre-diabetics had a 54 percent increase in heart attacks when compared to those with normal blood glucose levels!

The goal with type 2 diabetes is to convince your cells to respond again. If you treat them right by exercising, eating healthy foods, and losing weight, the cells can start functioning normally. Diabetes can be reversed if you work hard. A better solution is to control your risk factors and avoid diabetes altogether.

## NO. 7 KILLER: INFLUENZA AND PNEUMONIA— GET YOUR VACCINATION IF YOU'RE AT RISK

Here, finally, at number seven on the leading causes of death, are the first infectious diseases: the respiratory infections influenza and pneumonia, two of the most deadly diseases of past centuries. Influenza has gotten much more attention in recent years and could pose a serious threat if we are visited by a pandemic strain, such as the one that killed more than twenty million people in 1918. But year in and year out, pneumonia kills more than thirty times as many people as influenza, most of them elderly.

Pneumonia is an inflammation of the lung caused by infection from bacteria, viruses, and other organisms. It occurs when your immune system is weakened, especially if you are very young, elderly, or suffering from other diseases that lower resistance to infection. You should talk with your doctor to determine if you are a candidate for the pneumonia vaccination.

Influenza, or flu, is a respiratory infection caused by flu viruses. Fortunately, most people who get the flu are better within a week or so. For the very young, elderly, and those with chronic diseases, however, the flu and its complications, including pneumonia, can be life threatening.

The flu viruses are constantly changing, and different forms circulate each year. As a result,

### Major Risk Factors for Influenza and Pneumonia

▶ Age—the elderly and very young
▶ Tobacco use/lung disease
▶ Decreased immune function: AIDS, history of transplant, cancer treatment
▶ Chronic diseases, including cardiovascular disease, diabetes, cancer, congestive heart failure, and asthma
▶ History of splenectomy/ sickle cell anemia
▶ Lack of exercise

the formulation of the flu vaccine changes, and people who get vaccines need to get a new one each year, usually in the fall. Talk with your doctor to determine if you are a candidate for the influenza vaccine.

## NO. 8 KILLER: ALZHEIMER'S— A VASCULAR DISEASE?

Alzheimer's disease . . . the dreaded Alzheimer's. When we ask our patients what diseases they fear most, it's unquestionably Alzheimer's disease.

Alzheimer's disease, the eighth leading cause of death in the United States, is an insidious disorder that progressively ravages the brain, destroying a person's memory, intellect, and dignity. Alzheimer's disease takes away the ability to learn new things, make judgments, communicate, reason, and conduct daily activities. As the disease progresses, some people also suffer behavioral changes, such as anxiety, suspiciousness, delusions, and hallucinations.

Actress Kate Mulgrew, known for her portrayal of Captain Kathryn Janeway on the television show *Star Trek: Voyager* and a spokeswoman for the Alzheimer's Association, told an audience in Denver, "A lot of things happen when you turn fifty: your husband has a heart attack, you get hot flashes, and your mother, after pausing to take a good look at you, says, 'I like you, you are funny, but who are you?'"

Ms. Mulgrew went on to say, "Alzheimer's is not so much a disease as it is a tragedy. Death comes with an aching slowness, and the grief is almost unbearable." This sums up Alzheimer's disease as well as any statement we have ever heard.

Part of the tragedy is that people with Alzheimer's live so long with the disease. Patients live on average eight to ten years after diagnosis, and can live as long as twenty years with the disease. Alzheimer's disease kills about sixty-four thousand people in the United States every year. The number of people with Alzheimer's has doubled since 1980 to an estimated 4.5 million in the United States today, and it is expected to continue climbing as the Baby Boom generation ages.

Alzheimer's disease is not a normal part of aging. The brain cells of patients with Alzheimer's develop clumps and strands of proteins, known as amyloid plaques and neurofibrillary tangles, which kill the cells. No one knows if the plaques and tangles are a cause of Alzheimer's or a byproduct of another process.

Currently there is no cure for Alzheimer's disease. Some medications have been approved recently for treatment of the disease, but these medications have not proven particularly effective at warding off the symptoms, and they do nothing to cure the disease.

As far as prevention, keeping the brain sharp and healthy seems to be helpful. This is done by not smoking, eating a healthy diet, getting exercise, avoiding excessive alcohol, being socially active, and working the mind, such as doing crossword puzzles or reading. The research, however, is far from definitive about how to prevent Alzheimer's disease. In fact, we still don't even know its cause.

So why is Alzheimer's disease included in a longevity book?

Mounting evidence has identified a close relationship between Alzheimer's disease and cardiovascular disease. In fact, recent clinical studies have challenged the assumption that Alzheimer's is purely a disease of the brain cells. A number of experts now suspect that Alzheimer's disease is a vascular disease; in other words, it's related to the health of our blood vessels. The good news is that we know a host of ways to keep our blood vessels healthy.

Dr. Larry Sparks, a well-known and respected researcher at the Sun Health Research Institute in Sun City, Arizona, did some of the original animal studies linking diet to heart disease. But he didn't stop there. Further studies looked at the link between diet and the brain. Dr. Sparks fed rabbits diets that were high in cholesterol and

## Risk Factors for Alzheimer's Disease

KNOWN risk factors for Alzheimer's disease

- Age—The disease usually strikes people over the age of sixty. About 5 percent of men and women ages sixty-five to seventy-four have Alzheimer's, and almost half of people eighty-five and older may have the disease.
- Family history/genetics—If you have a parent or sibling with Alzheimer's, you are two to three times more likely to develop the disease than those with no family history.
- Previous head injury/brain trauma.
- Gender—Women are at a higher risk of developing Alzheimer's than men because they live longer.

EMERGING risk factors for Alzheimer's disease

- Cardiovascular disease/diabetes
- Lack of omega-3 fatty acids, antioxidants, fruits/vegetables/nuts
- High saturated fat/trans fat diet
- Obesity
- Lack of exercise
- High cholesterol
- High blood pressure

saturated fat, and then he examined their brains. He found that the brains of these rabbits were full of amyloid plaque, one of the markers of Alzheimer's disease. When the rabbits were put on a healthy diet (and some were placed on a cholesterol-lowering statin medication), the amyloid plaques actually shrank!

Dr. Sparks also looked at the link between Alzheimer's patients and statin drugs, which lower cholesterol. He studied ninety-eight individuals who were mildly to moderately affected with Alzheimer's disease. Some of these patients were started on a high dose of a statin. After twelve months, 53 percent of the Alzheimer's patients had stabilized or improved. According to Dr. Sparks, there was "clear clinical benefit" in both cognition and depression. In addition, two large studies, both with over seventy thousand individuals, reported a 63–77 percent decrease in Alzheimer's disease among people taking statin drugs.

Researchers at the Sun Health Research Institute also compared the main artery at the base of the brain, called the Circle of Willis, in Alzheimer's patients and non-Alzheimer's patients after they had died. The arteries of Alzheimer's patients were clogged, while the arteries of the non-Alzheimer's patients were not. Alzheimer's disease was clearly associated with decreased blood flow in the brain.

In an editorial that accompanied the Circle of Willis findings, Dr. Constantino Iadecola, of Cornell University's Weill Medical College, pointed out a number of important facts linking Alzheimer's and vascular disease. First, the risk factors for vascular disease, such as diabetes, high cholesterol, hypertension, poor diet, and lack of physical activity, are also risk factors for Alzheimer's disease. Second, symptoms of Alzheimer's disease are worse in people who have areas of decreased blood flow in their brains. Third, brain scans of asymptomatic patients who were merely at risk for Alzheimer's disease show marked alterations in cerebral blood flow.

Although this research is not conclusive, there is a growing body of evidence suggesting that Alzheimer's disease may result from atherosclerosis and decreased blood flow in the brain. It is exciting to think that we might be able to prevent Alzheimer's disease by doing the same proven things we use for heart disease—exercise, diet, and statin medications.

## NO. 9 KILLER: KIDNEY DISEASE

Although kidney disease is officially the ninth leading cause of death in the United States, it is even more serious than its ranking suggests; a majority of people with chronic kidney disease actually die of heart disease.

> **Risk Factors for Kidney Disease**
>
> ▸ Diabetes
> ▸ High blood pressure

The two main causes of chronic kidney disease are diabetes and high blood pressure, which are responsible for up to two-thirds of all cases. Diabetes is the leading cause of kidney failure. So, if you take a good look at the information on diabetes and high blood pressure in this book and concentrate on preventive practices, you can greatly reduce your risk for kidney disease.

## NO. 10 KILLER: SEPTICEMIA

Septicemia is a bacterial infection that begins in a localized area in the body, then enters the bloodstream and becomes widespread. The death rate from septicemia is an alarming 50 percent. Unfortunately, everyone is at potential risk of developing septicemia—even from minor infections or illnesses. However, the odds of getting septicemia are much greater if you have one or more of the risk factors.

> **Risk Factors for Septicemia**
>
> ▸ Very young or very old
> ▸ Weakened immune system
> ▸ Wounds, injuries, or burns
> ▸ Alcohol/drug abuse
> ▸ Intravenous catheters, wound drainage, urinary catheters
> ▸ Lack of proper vaccinations

Septicemia is not a preventable disease like some of the others mentioned in this book, but like all of the other diseases, it has preventive components. Taking good care of yourself, getting proper vaccinations, and keeping your immune system strong with exercise and nutritious foods are the best strategies for preventing infections and, thus, septicemia.

## CHAPTER 3

# Your Personal Risk Profile

Each person is unique. The specific combination of lifestyle, genetics, age, and other factors gives each of us our own personal health profile. Some of these factors give us a better chance of living a long and healthy life, while others put us at risk for developing the common diseases we reviewed in the last chapter. These elements are known as risk factors.

In order to take advantage of the longevity advice in this book, you need to know your risk factors. They will help you identify which of the top ten diseases are most likely to rob you of health and longevity. Below is a list of the eleven most common and important risk factors, with basic benchmarks to help you decide which ones are risk factors for you.

Once you have finished this chapter, you will be able to create your own personal risk profile. Then, you can focus your efforts on controlling, reducing, and monitoring the risk factors that pose the greatest threat to your chances of living a long and healthy life.

## Common Risk Factors for the Ten Most Deadly Diseases

**Controllable risk factors**

High cholesterol
Poor diet
High blood pressure
Tobacco use
Sedentary lifestyle/lack of regular exercise
Overweight/obesity
Too much alcohol

**Uncontrollable risk factors**

Genetics
Age
Gender
Race

# RISK FACTOR NO. 1: WHAT'S YOUR CHOLESTEROL?

Back in 1979, the World Health Organization took a look at heart disease on a global scale. The country with the lowest per capita rate of heart disease was Japan. The country with the highest rate—ten times that of Japan—was Finland.

Why, you may ask, was there such a difference? According to the World Health Organization, the single biggest cause of heart disease and one of the culprits for the dramatically different rates of heart disease in Finland and Japan was cholesterol.

In Japan the average total cholesterol in 1979 was 140 milligrams per deciliter (mg/dL). In Finland it was 280 mg/dL. The United States, with an average cholesterol level of 260, was the third highest for both cholesterol and heart disease, just behind Scotland.

The good news is that between 1979 and 1992, Finland reduced the number of deaths due to heart disease and strokes by a huge 55

## Mortality from Coronary Artery Disease and Cholesterol, 1979

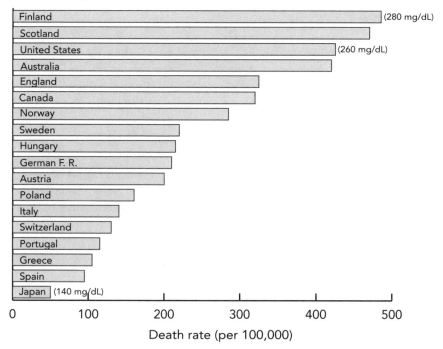

*In 1979, countries with the highest average cholesterol levels also had the highest rates of death from coronary artery disease.* (*Source:* Osmo Turpeinen, MD, PhD, "Effect of cholesterol-lowering diet on mortality from coronary heart disease and other causes," *Circulation* 59 [1979], 1–7.)

percent! About 80 percent of this decline was attributed to an emphasis on recognizing and reducing the major risk factors: smoking, high cholesterol, and high blood pressure. Of those, a significant drop in cholesterol level was the largest contributor to reducing heart disease death in Finland.

Cholesterol is a soft, waxy substance that comes from two sources. It is made in the liver and also comes from foods we consume, especially egg yolks, meat, and whole-fat dairy products. Cholesterol is crucial for a healthy body; it is an essential part of cell walls, skin, and the lining of nerves.

## Components of Cholesterol

Cholesterol is made up of HDL, LDL, and triglycerides. Your total cholesterol number is important, but your readings on each of these components provides valuable information as well. HDL is the "good" cholesterol, so you want this number to be high; LDL is the "bad" cholesterol, so you want this number to be low. Triglycerides, the chemical form in which fat exists in the body, should also be low.

LDL stands for low-density lipoprotein, which refers to a class of lipoprotein particles, varying in size and content, that transport cholesterol in the blood stream from the liver to cells throughout the body. Too much LDL-cholesterol is associated with an increased risk of developing heart disease and stroke.

HDL, or high-density lipoprotein, helps transport excess artery-blocking cholesterol out of the bloodstream and into the liver. It eventually leaves the body through the gastrointestinal system.

Unlike LDL levels, which are often a result of diet and heredity, HDL levels are linked more to one's lifestyle than to diet alone. Smoking, obesity, and lack of physical activity are directly linked to low blood HDL levels. Accordingly, weight loss, smoking cessation, and exercise will raise HDL levels.

Controlling total cholesterol is a combination of raising the good and lowering the bad, which is accomplished with both dietary and lifestyle changes. However, sometimes lifestyle modification and diet alone are not enough to reach recommended cholesterol levels. In these cases, medication may be necessary.

Triglycerides are the molecules the body uses to store fat, and they are another "bad" component of the cholesterol profile. Calories consumed during a meal that are not used immediately are converted to triglycerides and transported to fat cells to be stored. Most triglycerides are found in fat tissue. Some triglycerides circulate in the blood to provide fuel for muscles to work. Either way, you want your triglyceride numbers to be low. Excess triglycerides in the bloodstream are linked to coronary artery disease, and, like LDL, triglycerides can also deposit themselves along the walls of arteries, contributing to plaque, which leads to atherosclerosis.

## Genetics and Cholesterol

| | Cholesterol Level (mg/dL) | Incidence | Age When Heart Disease Develops |
|---|---|---|---|
| Familial hypercholesteremia (two genes) | Above 800 | 1 in 1,000,000 | 13–19 |
| Familial hypercholesteremia (one gene) | 300–400 | 1 in 500 | 31–55 |
| Average American | 215 (200–300) | 3 in 4 | 60s |
| Good | Below 200 | 1 in 5 | 70+ |
| Optimal | 150 | 1 in 20 | almost never |

*Sources:* William C. Roberts, MD, "Atherosclerotic risk factors—are there ten or is there only one?" *The American Journal of Cardiology* 64 (September 1, 1989), 552–555; William P. Castelli, MD, "Making practical sense of clinical trial data in decreasing cardiovascular risk," *The American Journal of Cardiology* 88 (August 16, 2001), 16–20.

But too much cholesterol can lead to heart disease. This excess of cholesterol, usually from dietary intake, is deposited in the arteries and causes fatty buildup inside blood vessels, a process called atherosclerosis. Atherosclerosis narrows the blood vessels, restricts blood flow, and creates perfect spots for blood clots to form, completely blocking blood flow. A heart attack occurs when blood flow is blocked in the vessels of the heart.

Since 1948, researchers have been studying thousands of people in Framingham, Massachusetts, to learn more about heart disease, including its prevention and risk factors. In fact, many of the landmark scientific papers that have been published about heart disease in America have been based on the Framingham Heart Study. A former lead researcher of this study, Dr. William Castelli, noted, "In forty years, we never found a heart attack in anyone with cholesterol below 150." He went on to say, "Close to 90 percent of all coronary death could be prevented if the cholesterol was kept below 182 mg/dL, blood pressure under 120 mmHg, and no smoking or diabetes."

## Cholesterol—Lifestyle, Not Genetics

A compelling research study that looked at cholesterol levels among Japanese immigrants helped us to understand the relationship between diet and lifestyle and our risk of developing heart disease. This study followed middle-aged Japanese men who had migrated to Honolulu and then to California. The average cholesterol of Japanese men living in Japan was 140 mg/dL, while the average cholesterol of the Japanese who moved to Hawaii increased to 200 mg/dL in just a few short years.

Then, the researchers looked at those Japanese immigrants who left Hawaii and moved to Los Angeles. Well, it's probably not hard for you to believe that their average cholesterol shot up to 250 mg/dL! Clearly, high cholesterol is not a genetic thing. Unfortunately, it's the American diet and lifestyle that caused this dramatic increase.

Dr. William Roberts, editor of *The American Journal of Cardiology*, looked at the ten risk factors for heart disease that were identified by the National Cholesterol Education Program. These risk factors include elevated cholesterol, definitive evidence of coronary artery disease, gender, family history, cigarette smoking, hypertension, diabetes, cerebrovascular or peripheral vascular disease, and severe obesity. Roberts states that "the only *absolute* prerequisite for a fatal or nonfatal atherosclerotic event is a serum total cholesterol level greater than 150 mg/dL."

There is also evidence that high cholesterol is a significant factor in several other diseases, including stroke, Alzheimer's disease, kidney disease, eye disease, and peripheral vascular disease. This makes sense because cholesterol affects all blood vessels, not just those in the heart.

**Cholesterol Benchmark:**

▸ *Total cholesterol: under 200 mg/dL; optimal under 150 mg/dL*

▸ *HDL: more than 45 mg/dL; optimal more than 50 mg/dL*

▸ *LDL: less than 100 mg/dL; optimal 70 mg/dL if you have a history of heart attack, stroke, other vascular disease, or diabetes*

▸ *Triglycerides: under 150 mg/dL, optimal under 100 mg/dL*

▸ *Total cholesterol/HDL ratio: less than 3.5, optimally less than 3.0*


## RISK FACTOR NO. 2:
## POOR DIET—WE ARE WHAT WE EAT

The 1979 World Health Organization study that highlighted the impact of cholesterol on heart disease also highlighted the importance of diet. It started with an interesting observation: deaths from heart disease dropped significantly during the Second World War in Finland and Norway when many of the foods high in saturated fat—meat and dairy products especially—were in short supply. When the war was over and the food supply returned to its previous levels, so did deaths from heart disease. The study went on to show definitively that diets high in saturated fat are associated with high cholesterol levels and a greater incidence of heart disease.

We have also learned that many cancers are related to a poor diet. We know that eating lots of fruits and vegetables can decrease our risk of cancer. And it's obvious that overeating leads to obesity and type 2 diabetes. All of these diseases are related to personal choices that we make about what and how much to eat. We need to be better about connecting the dots and recognizing the relationship between our eating habits and our diseases.

## Herbivores or Carnivores: Are Humans Confused?

Cats and dogs are carnivores—they are designed to eat meat. Orang-utans are herbivores—they do not eat meat. If you put a Big Mac in an orangutan's cage, he will eat the sesame seed bun, the lettuce, tomato, pickle and special sauce, but he will not touch the all-beef patty. In contrast, if you put a Big Mac in a lion's cage, he will eat the all-beef patty and leave the bun, pickle, tomato, and lettuce.

There are large physiologic differences between herbivores and carnivores. One of the most fascinating differences between the two (and it may not seem to make sense at first) is that carnivores don't get atherosclerosis and herbivores do.

Which do you think you are? It just so happens that humans—*homo sapiens*—share the characteristics of the herbivores, such as flat molars, lack of claws, weak stomach acids, and long intestinal tracks. But most of us conduct our lives as if we were omnivores, eating meat as well as vegetables and fruits. Since we are designed as herbivores, not carnivores, we get atherosclerosis (unlike our family cat or dog).

We're not saying you can't eat meat. Meat is a good source of protein, zinc, and iron, but too much of it can also be detrimental to your health. The key to a healthy diet lies in knowing what to eat and making the right choices. We recommend consuming a mostly vegetarian diet, with occasional lean cuts of meat.

What should we eat? On the next page is a basic guideline for a healthy diet. Chapter 5 offers even more information on "super-foods," simple suggestions for eating better, and ways to cut down on the amount of food you eat. We have also listed healthy recipes in the appendix.

**Carnivores vs. Herbivores**

|  | Carnivores | Herbivores |
|---|---|---|
| Appendages | Claws | Hand/hoof |
| Teeth | Sharp (for ripping) | Flat (for grinding) |
| Intestinal tract | Short (rapid digestion) | Long (for nutrient absorption) |
| Body cooling | Panting | Sweating |
| Method of drinking | Lapping | Sipping |
| Vitamin C | Make their own | Obtain from diet |
| Stomach acid | 20x | 1x |
| Can develop atherosclerosis | No | Yes |

Source: William C. Roberts, MD, "Atherosclerosis: Its cause and its prevention," *The American Journal of Cardiology* 98 (December 1, 2006), 1550–1555.

## Diet Benchmark:

▸ *A variety of fruits and vegetables, at least five servings a day, preferably nine. Choose those with bright, deep colors for better antioxidant and polyphenol properties.*

▸ *Whole grains, such as whole wheat, brown rice, and oatmeal*

▸ *Fish several times a week, particularly salmon, sardines, tuna, trout, and herring*

▸ *Legumes, including soy, beans, peas, and lentils*

▸ *Lean meats*

▸ *Nuts*

▸ *Low-fat dairy products*

▸ *Foods low in saturated fat, trans fat, and cholesterol*

▸ *Limited salt*

▸ *Minimal sugary, processed foods (cookies, soda, candy)*

▸ *Alcoholic beverages: one-to-two per day*

## RISK FACTOR NO. 3: DO YOU HAVE HYPERTENSION?

Have you ever seen the devastating effects of a heavy rainstorm and flooding? A large volume of water flowing at high pressure has the power to wear down concrete walls and erode the foundations of homes. Well, the blood flow of people with high blood pressure, also known as hypertension, is quite similar. When blood flows through your arteries at a high pressure for a long time, it damages the fragile layer of cells lining the arteries, called the endothelium. This is how hypertension contributes to heart disease.

When high blood pressure damages the endothelium, lipids from the blood can easily enter the injured artery wall, leading to the formation of foam cells, fatty streaks, and, eventually, a huge, ugly plaque. So, high blood pressure actually accelerates the process of atherosclerosis.

Hypertension doesn't just affect the heart, however. In addition to causing atherosclerosis, which can lead to heart attacks and strokes, hypertension damages blood vessels throughout the body, leading to limb amputations, kidney disease, heart failure, and blindness.

The cause of hypertension is elusive. We know that a small percentage of hypertension cases are associated with kidney and adrenal disease. And we know that being overweight, smoking, and using excessive salt in your diet can contribute to high blood pressure. But we cannot directly identify the primary cause of high blood pressure in 95 percent of cases. We do know, however, that blood pressure needs to be controlled.

Blood pressure has two readings: systolic, the top number, and diastolic, the bottom number. Blood pressure of 120/80 millimeters of mercury (mm Hg) is considered good, while 140/90 has historically been considered the threshold for "high" blood pressure, a situation that needs attention.

## Hypertension—A Presidential Story

The final years of Franklin D. Roosevelt painfully illuminate the enormous progress we have made in treating high blood pressure.

In *The Dying President: Franklin D. Roosevelt, 1944–1945,* author Robert H. Ferrell reviews Roosevelt's medical history, including the former president's blood pressure readings from the time he was vice president in 1931 (140/90) to the morning of his death on April 12, 1945, when it was 300+/190.

At 12:45 p.m. on his final day, FDR suffered a hemorrhagic stroke, and at 3:35 p.m., fewer than three hours later, while his doctor stood by helplessly, he was pronounced dead.

Only sixty years ago we had no reliable treatment for high blood pressure. Since then, we have made amazing medical progress. What happened to FDR (untreated malignant hypertension) should *not* happen today.

However, doctors with the Framingham Heart Study showed that even high-normal blood pressure of 130–139/85–89 increased a woman's chances of developing cardiovascular disease by 60 percent and a man's chances by 150 percent over a ten-year period.

Another significant research project that changed national guidelines on blood pressure analyzed the findings of sixty-one separate studies, totaling one million adults, which made it one of the largest studies ever conducted in the field of medicine. Published in 2002, the study demonstrated that a twenty-point increase in your systolic blood pressure doubles your risk of heart attack or stroke. Heart attacks increase eightfold as blood pressure goes from 120 to 180, and stroke increases by thirteenfold! You can cut your risk of heart attack or stroke in half by dropping your blood pressure twenty points.

Get your blood pressure checked regularly, anywhere and every chance you get—at pharmacies, supermarkets, and health fairs. Make sure it is normal, 120/80. If it isn't, do something to lower it: exercise, change your diet, and take medication, if needed. Don't take chances. Lowering blood pressure is essential to your health and longevity.

**Blood Pressure Benchmark:**

▸ *120/80 millimeters of mercury*

## RISK FACTOR NO. 4: TOBACCO USE— THE SINGLE MOST PREVENTABLE CAUSE OF DEATH

Every cigarette takes an average of seven minutes off your life. The U.S. Centers for Disease Control and Prevention estimates that adult male smokers lose an average of 13.2 years of life and female smokers lose 14.5 years of life. Smoking is responsible for more than half a million deaths every year in the United States and accounts for one out of every five deaths nationally. These deaths are preventable. In fact, smoking has been identified as *the single most preventable cause of death and disease in the United States!*

According to the American Cancer Society, smoking has been linked to at least ten different types of cancer, and it accounts for up to 30 percent of all cancer deaths. What most people don't know, however, is that more smokers die of heart disease than of cancer. In fact, smoking is a contributing factor in up to 40 percent of all deaths due to cardiovascular disease. In addition, smoking is the major cause of chronic obstructive pulmonary disease (COPD), the fourth leading cause of death in the United States.

If you live in a household where others smoke, or work in a smoky environment, you face an elevated risk of developing diseases associated with tobacco. Secondhand smoke measurably increases the risk of lung cancer, and it has also been shown to increase the risk of coronary artery disease and stroke in nonsmokers.

Cigar and pipe smoking also increase the risk of coronary artery disease, COPD, and cancers of the mouth, neck, esophagus, and lung. Smokeless tobacco users have a greater risk of heart disease than do those who use no tobacco at all.

**Tobacco Benchmark:**
> ▸ *Avoid all forms of tobacco and tobacco smoke*

## RISK FACTOR NO. 5: LACK OF EXERCISE

In the previous chapter we pointed out that lack of exercise is a risk factor for five of the top ten most deadly diseases. But, in reality, getting enough exercise can improve your chances of avoiding *all* of those diseases, from cancer to accidents to infections. (See sidebar on page 46 "Exercise Helps Prevent All of the Top Ten Diseases.")

Exercise does *all the right things* for your body and mind. It helps you lose weight; strengthens your heart, bones, and lungs; and improves your mood, health, and longevity.

There are hundreds of thousands of medications available today to treat your various ailments. But there's not a single medication that delivers all the beneficial effects you can get from exercise. Exercise will prevent disease, it will improve your disease, and, in some cases, exercise will cure your disease. But you have to do it. Don't let your body down.

**Exercise Benchmark:**
> ▸ *Exercise for at least thirty minutes every day. Period, no excuses.*

## Exercise Helps Prevent All of the Top Ten Diseases

**Heart disease:** Exercise lowers cholesterol levels, reduces inflammation, and decreases the risk of clotting. Abundant evidence definitively shows that exercise prevents the development of coronary artery disease and reduces the symptoms in patients with established coronary disease.

**Cancer:** The 2006 "American Cancer Society Guidelines on Nutrition and Physical Activity for Cancer Prevention" includes ample evidence that exercise can reduce your risk of cancer, particularly colon and breast cancer.

**Stroke:** Exercise helps lower blood pressure and, therefore, lowers the likelihood of stroke and kidney disease. Many studies show that exercise may be all that is needed to control blood pressure in some mildly hypertensive people.

**Lung disease:** The majority of deaths due to lung cancer are related to the effects of smoking cigarettes. Studies have shown that people who exercise are twice as likely as sedentary people to successfully quit smoking.

**Accidents:** Exercise helps reduce your risk of dying from falls, an increasing problem in our aging population. Exercise keeps your bones strong and your body more flexible. It improves balance, and it helps your body respond more quickly to dangerous situations.

**Diabetes:** There is indisputable evidence that exercise decreases the onset of diabetes, improves metabolic syndrome, improves carbohydrate metabolism, decreases obesity, and improves insulin sensitivity. The Diabetes Prevention Program, a major research study, demonstrated that physical activity, combined with weight loss, reduced the onset of type 2 diabetes by 58 percent over a twenty-eight-year period. This was more effective than medication, which reduced the onset by 31 percent.

**Influenza, pneumonia, and septicemia:** Exercise improves our immune system and helps us fight off infections.

**Alzheimer's disease:** Exercise improves cognitive function and helps to decrease the ravages of Alzheimer's disease.

**Kidney disease:** As noted above, exercise helps reduce hypertension, heart disease, and diabetes, the three leading causes of kidney disease.

## RISK FACTOR NO. 6: EXCESS WEIGHT AND OBESITY

We've all seen the headlines about the obesity epidemic in this country. But did you know that two-thirds of adults over twenty can be categorized as overweight? With 300 million people in this country, it is sobering to realize that 200 million of us are an unhealthy weight.

There was a cartoon circulating recently that featured an overweight bride and groom looking at their three-tiered wedding cake. The bride says to the groom, "We have sixty guests and only three pieces of cake!" Clearly, we have very relaxed attitudes these days about overeating and being "super-sized."

The U.S. Centers for Disease Control and Prevention published a revealing map of obesity in the United States. In 1991, in the four fattest states in the country, 15–19 percent of the population was obese, with a body mass index of greater than thirty. By 2004, however, an obesity rate of 15–19 percent qualified seven states not as the fattest but as the leanest ones in the nation. In nine states more than a quarter of the population was obese—not just overweight, but obese! Those are scary numbers. What's going to happen in the next ten years?

### What the extra pounds do to your health

Being overweight or obese is a risk factor for cardiovascular disease, hypertension, and high cholesterol, as well as a significant risk factor for developing type 2 diabetes. Obesity is also associated with more than thirty other medical conditions, including gallbladder disease, sleep apnea, arthritis, and several forms of cancer (breast, esophagus, colorectal, endometrial, and renal cell). Furthermore, obesity can complicate the treatment and management of these and other conditions.

| Height (in.) | | | | | | Body Weight (pounds) | | | | | | | | | | |
|---|---|---|---|---|---|---|---|---|---|---|---|---|---|---|---|---|
| | Normal Weight | | | | | Overweight | | | | | Obese | | | | | |
| 58 | 91 | 96 | 100 | 105 | 110 | 115 | 119 | 124 | 129 | 134 | 138 | 143 | 148 | 153 | 158 | 162 | 167 |
| 59 | 94 | 99 | 104 | 109 | 114 | 119 | 124 | 128 | 133 | 138 | 143 | 148 | 153 | 158 | 163 | 168 | 173 |
| 60 | 97 | 102 | 107 | 112 | 118 | 123 | 128 | 133 | 138 | 143 | 148 | 153 | 158 | 163 | 168 | 174 | 179 |
| 61 | 100 | 106 | 111 | 116 | 122 | 127 | 132 | 137 | 143 | 148 | 153 | 158 | 164 | 169 | 174 | 180 | 185 |
| 62 | 104 | 109 | 115 | 120 | 126 | 131 | 136 | 142 | 147 | 153 | 158 | 164 | 169 | 175 | 180 | 186 | 191 |
| 63 | 107 | 113 | 118 | 124 | 130 | 135 | 141 | 146 | 152 | 158 | 163 | 169 | 175 | 180 | 186 | 191 | 197 |
| 64 | 110 | 116 | 122 | 128 | 134 | 140 | 145 | 151 | 157 | 163 | 169 | 174 | 180 | 186 | 192 | 197 | 204 |
| 65 | 114 | 120 | 126 | 132 | 138 | 144 | 150 | 156 | 162 | 168 | 174 | 180 | 186 | 192 | 198 | 204 | 210 |
| 66 | 118 | 124 | 130 | 136 | 142 | 148 | 155 | 161 | 167 | 173 | 179 | 186 | 192 | 198 | 204 | 210 | 216 |
| 67 | 121 | 127 | 134 | 140 | 146 | 153 | 159 | 166 | 172 | 178 | 185 | 191 | 198 | 204 | 211 | 217 | 223 |
| 68 | 125 | 131 | 138 | 144 | 151 | 158 | 164 | 171 | 177 | 184 | 190 | 197 | 203 | 210 | 216 | 223 | 230 |
| 69 | 128 | 135 | 142 | 149 | 155 | 162 | 169 | 176 | 182 | 189 | 196 | 203 | 209 | 216 | 223 | 230 | 236 |
| 70 | 132 | 139 | 146 | 153 | 160 | 167 | 174 | 181 | 188 | 195 | 202 | 209 | 216 | 222 | 229 | 236 | 243 |
| 71 | 136 | 143 | 150 | 157 | 165 | 172 | 179 | 186 | 193 | 200 | 208 | 215 | 222 | 229 | 236 | 243 | 250 |
| 72 | 140 | 147 | 154 | 162 | 169 | 177 | 184 | 191 | 199 | 206 | 213 | 221 | 228 | 235 | 242 | 250 | 258 |
| 73 | 144 | 151 | 159 | 166 | 174 | 182 | 189 | 197 | 204 | 212 | 219 | 227 | 235 | 242 | 250 | 257 | 265 |
| 74 | 148 | 155 | 163 | 171 | 179 | 186 | 194 | 202 | 210 | 218 | 225 | 233 | 241 | 249 | 256 | 264 | 272 |
| 75 | 152 | 160 | 168 | 176 | 184 | 192 | 200 | 208 | 216 | 224 | 232 | 240 | 248 | 256 | 264 | 272 | 279 |
| 76 | 156 | 164 | 172 | 180 | 189 | 197 | 205 | 213 | 221 | 230 | 238 | 246 | 254 | 263 | 271 | 279 | 287 |
| BMI | 19 | 20 | 21 | 22 | 23 | 24 | 25 | 26 | 27 | 28 | 29 | 30 | 31 | 32 | 33 | 34 | 35 |

Source: National Heart, Lung, and Blood Institute.

### What's your BMI?

Body mass index (BMI) is a fancy way to tell you if you are overweight or obese. (Although you can usually tell just by looking in the mirror.) It is calculated as your weight (converted into kilograms) divided by your height (converted into meters) squared. Rather than do those laborious calculations, you can look at the table above to determine your BMI.

BMI Benchmark:
▸ *Body mass index (BMI) of 25 or less*

## Major Conditions Associated with Obesity

- Arthritis
- Birth defects
- Cancer
- Cardiovascular disease
- Carpal tunnel syndrome
- Chronic venous insufficiency
- Daytime sleepiness
- Deep vein thrombosis
- End stage renal disease
- Gallbladder disease
- Gout
- Heart disorders
- Impaired immune response
- Impaired respiratory function
- Incontinence
- Infections following wounds
- Infertility
- Liver disease
- Low back pain
- Pancreatitis
- Sleep apnea
- Stroke
- Surgical complications
- Type 2 diabetes

### And your waist size?

Another important measurement that is a good predictor of health risk is abdominal fat. Those with an increased waist circumference are at an increased risk for developing type 2 diabetes, cholesterol disorders, high blood pressure, and cardiovascular disease.

**Waist-Size Benchmark:**
- *For men, a waist circumference smaller than forty inches*
- *For women, a waist circumference smaller than thirty-five inches*

## RISK FACTOR NO. 7: ALCOHOL—A LITTLE IS GOOD, BUT TOO MUCH IS TERRIBLE

There have been more than seventy major reports, state-of-the-art papers, science advisories, and scientific statements that describe the benefit of mild-to-moderate alcohol intake in preventing cardiovascular disease.

Overall, all types of cardiovascular disease (coronary artery disease, strokes, heart failure, peripheral vascular disease) appear to benefit from drinking small amounts of daily alcohol. It is also beneficial for improved lipids, especially raising HDL, decreased clotting, reduced inflammation, and improved insulin response.

However, we cannot overlook the detrimental effects of overconsumption of alcohol. It ruins lives, careers, and marriages, and has adverse affects on a fetus, a child, or a loved one. Too much alcohol also ruins your health, leading to hypertension, stroke, arrhythmias, sudden death, cancer, cirrhosis, automobile accidents, trauma, homicides, suicides, addiction, and increased risk of breast cancer. Remember, one to two drinks a day have health benefits. Anything more is bad for your health.

**Alcohol Benchmark:**
- *One drink per day for women*
- *One to two drinks per day for men*
- *A drink is defined as twelve ounces of beer, five ounces of wine, or one and a half ounces of spirits*


## UNCONTROLLABLE RISK FACTORS

The previous seven risk factors are ones that you can control: you can change your diet, lower your blood pressure, and get exercise.

The following four risk factors, however, are uncontrollable; you can't change your genetics, age, race, or gender. So, if you can't do anything about them, then why put them in this book? Because if you know the threats that these various risk factors pose, you can monitor your health more closely with the screening tests we recommend in Chapter 10. Then, you can take steps to counter their ill effects by making extra efforts to reduce your controllable risk factors and to take medications, if needed.

## RISK FACTOR NO. 8: GENETICS

Do you have "nice genes?" An internationally acclaimed lipid specialist, Dr. Robert Vogel, was in southern France on a trip with friends when he looked up to see if he was going in the right direction. He laughed out loud at what he saw. There was a sign with an arrow pointing toward the cities Nice and Genes. It made him think about the genetics of heart disease. Do you have "nice genes"? Have you chosen your parents wisely? Is heart disease a genetic problem?

Many patients come to us and lament the fact that heart disease runs in their family. They feel as if they are doomed to the same fate as their parents. We often reply, "It's not the disease you inherit from your parents, it's their bad habits!"

We have scrutinized the data and have found that the overwhelming majority of heart disease can be clearly explained by controllable risk factors, not by genetics. What we inherit from our parents are not harmful genes, but their harmful habits.

This is not to say that there is no genetic component to heart disease. There is. In fact, there are about twenty to thirty genetic disorders that can cause heart disease, but these account for only 5 to 10 percent of patients. More than 90 percent of heart disease is caused by controllable risk factors.

Heart disease is like most of the other diseases on the top ten list. While genes do play a role in who gets disease, they generally have a much smaller impact than most people believe. For example, about 10–15 percent of cancers have a hereditary component, with breast cancer, colon cancer, and ovarian cancer more likely to have genetic origins. Scientists have also identified a gene that increases the chances of developing Alzheimer's disease.

So, people may have genes that predispose them to a specific disease, but they would rarely develop the disease without the contribution of unhealthy lifestyles. Genes alone are almost never enough to cause any of the ten most deadly diseases.

In general, though, if close family members, such as a mother, father, grandparent, or sibling, developed one of the diseases, you may have a higher risk of developing it yourself. You should make an extra effort to control any risk factors that contribute to the disease and talk to your doctor about getting screening tests to detect early signs of the disease.

## RISK FACTOR NO. 9: AGE

Increasing age is a risk factor for most of the top ten diseases. Heart disease and Alzheimer's disease are especially diseases of the elderly. Half of all people over the age of sixty die of heart disease, as do 70 percent of those over seventy-five.

The risk of developing Alzheimer's disease starts at age sixty-five and doubles every five years after that. By age eighty-five, the risk reaches nearly 50 percent.

But just because you are getting older doesn't mean you shouldn't control your risk factors for heart disease and Alzheimer's disease. You should be vigilant about risk factors at any age.

## Prevention Works among the Elderly

Too often, the elderly are underserved and undertreated. Many elderly patients and their doctors don't think that current medical guidelines pertain to this age group. But that is not true; the elderly are entitled to the same prevention tools as the rest of the population. In fact, when properly treated, older people have better prevention results than those who are less than seventy years of age. In a presentation at the American College of Cardiology in March 2005, Harvard researchers described a study in which they looked at individuals over age seventy with high and low LDL cholesterol levels. There were 75 percent fewer heart attacks in the group with lower LDL levels. In our practice, we let our elderly patients decide how aggressive they want to be. Not surprisingly, most of our elderly patients want to prevent strokes and heart attacks just as much as our younger patients do.

## RISK FACTOR NO. 10: GENDER

Men and women face different risks for different diseases. You should be aware of these differences so that you can take extra steps to protect yourself from the diseases that threaten you more, based on your gender.

You should also be aware of misperceptions about which diseases strike men or women more frequently. Heart disease is a prime example. Many people believe that men suffer heart disease more than women. The truth, in fact, is that more women than men die from heart disease. Cardiovascular disease is the leading cause of mortality for women in the United States. And, according to the American Heart Association, not only do more women die from heart disease than men, but the incidence of heart disease in women is increasing. Consider these sobering facts:

▸ Women have worse outcomes from heart attacks.
▸ Women have a greater recurrence of heart attacks.
▸ Women have less favorable outcomes after bypass surgery.
▸ Women have less frequent referrals for evaluation.
▸ Women have smaller arteries, which are harder to repair.
▸ Up to 40 percent of initial cardiac events in women are fatal!

Please remind the important women in your life that this disease is not to be minimized. It is as serious, if not more serious, in women

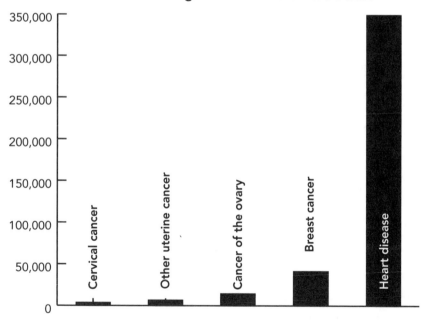

**Annual Deaths Among Women in the United States**

*Although heart disease gets less attention than breast and other female cancers, it poses a vastly greater threat to women's health in the United States* (*Source:* U.S. Centers for Disease Control and Prevention, "National Vital Statistics Reports," 54, no. 13 [April 19, 2006].)

as it is in men. Hence, our recommendations about heart disease throughout this book pertain to men and women alike.

Women also die more frequently from stroke; of every five deaths from stroke, two occur in men and three in women.

Slightly more men than women die of cancer, with tobacco-related cancers killing men more frequently. This rate is related to the historical pattern of men smoking in greater numbers, but that pattern is quickly changing. Expect women to catch up in tobacco-related cancers in the coming years.

Women have already caught up in the other smoking-related disease, chronic obstructive pulmonary disease (COPD). In just the past decade, women overtook men in the rate of death from COPD, although the figures are very close. However, this really has nothing to do with gender, and everything to do with who smokes.

Alzheimer's disease strikes men and women at about the same rate. But because Alzheimer's disease becomes increasingly common as people age, and because more women live longer than men, almost two-and-a-half times more women die of Alzheimer's disease than do men.

Almost twice as many men die in accidents, including motor vehicle accidents, nontransport accidents, accidental poisonings, and exposures to noxious substances. Men and women are about even in deaths caused by falls. Although they are not in the top ten most deadly diseases, suicide and assault also account for about four times as many deaths among men as among women.


## RISK FACTOR NO. 11: RACE

We have listed race as a risk factor in some diseases. However, the scientific literature is murky on whether the heightened risk is a result of biological or cultural factors. For example, heart disease is definitely higher among African Americans, although it's uncertain whether this increased rate is a result of a genetic predisposition or cultural influences, which may include a high-fat diet and limited exercise. Regardless of whether the heightened risk comes from biology or cultural practices, you should make sure you get plenty of exercise, avoid tobacco, eat balanced meals, and talk with your physician about your specific risk factors.

## CHAPTER 4

# Exercise:
# The Real Fountain of Youth

Exercise does all the right things for the biochemistry, the body, and the mind. Exercise lowers your weight, improves blood pressure dramatically, and increases energy. The benefits to heart, muscle, bones, and lungs have been exceedingly well established. Scientists are now coming to understand all the nuances of how exercise affects the body's inner workings and how it benefits so many separate systems.

## THE BIOCHEMISTRY OF EXERCISE

Exercise improves all cholesterol numbers. It is highly effective at raising the good cholesterol, or HDL. Furthermore, exercise dramatically lowers triglycerides, a form of fat found in your blood, and lowers the bad cholesterol, or LDL. In one noteworthy study, researchers demonstrated that people with a lower fitness level had higher cho-

lesterol and blood pressure, as well as lower levels of HDL cholesterol, than those in good physical shape.

In addition to improving cholesterol levels, exercise has a positive
effect on other biochemical markers associated with increased risk
of heart disease. Exercise can reduce inflammation in the arteries, a
well-known contributor to heart disease. Exercise also decreases
platelet stickiness, thus reducing the likelihood of developing artery-
blocking clots.

C-reactive protein in the blood has recently become recognized as
an important marker of inflammation, including inflammation in
the arteries. One study found that sedentary adults with high C-
reactive protein levels could lower those levels with a controlled exercise program. This finding may partly explain the effectiveness of
regular physical activity in the prevention and treatment of cardiovascular and metabolic diseases.

## THE MIND

Psychologists recommend exercise to improve self-esteem and self-
image. Exercise raises levels of the "feel-good" hormones, called en-
dorphins. It decreases anxiety and improves self-control and
attitude. Exercise helps us sleep more soundly and even helps allevi-
ate depression.

There is also exciting new evidence that exercise may improve
cognitive function and thinking, and delay or even prevent the onset
of dementia. In a comprehensive review of the existing medical literature, researchers Arthur Kramer, Kirk Erickson, and Stanley Colcombe, of the University of Illinois, found a significant relationship
between physical activity, better cognitive function, and decreased
occurrence of dementia, such as Alzheimer's disease. According to
Dr. Kramer, "We have found that physical and aerobic exercise train-

ing can lower the risk for developing some undesirable age-related changes in cognitive and brain functions, and also help the brain maintain its plasticity—its ability to cover one function if another starts failing later in life."

A person's reasoning and memory naturally decline with age. However, many studies have shown that improving cardiovascular fitness through exercise helps reduce and slow this decline. One especially encouraging study, which followed almost six thousand women over age sixty-five for at least six years, demonstrated that those who walked regularly had a lower chance of experiencing significant cognitive decline. Clearly, the benefits of regular exercise have no age limit. So don't use age as an excuse for not exercising!

## THE BODY: EXERCISE IS THE "FOUNTAIN OF YOUTH"

In fact, regular exercise becomes particularly important after the age of seventy. Between the ages of twenty and seventy, our aerobic capacity slowly declines at a rate of about 6 percent per decade. But after seventy, our bodies rapidly deteriorate, especially without exercise. The Baltimore Longitudinal Study of Aging points out that after age seventy, the body declines even in physically fit and active people at a rate of 20 percent per decade.

Now, here's the trouble that many elderly people face: they are in poor shape when they reach age seventy, but still don't make any lifestyle changes to counter this rapid physical decline. Consequently, they are frail, decrepit, and prone to all sorts of aging complications by the time they reach eighty. Their bodies are too weak to fight off infections, to survive a fall, or to recover after a heart attack or stroke.

On the other hand, a fit seventy-year-old can be in better shape than the average college student. Take, for example, oxygen consumption, which is a good measure of cardiovascular fitness. A seventy-year-old individual in excellent physical condition consumes about 38 milliliters of oxygen per kilogram of weight per minute (ml/kg/min) when running hard on a treadmill. In contrast, a twenty-year-old in average shape consumes about 33 ml/kg/min when doing the same activity. So, a fit seventy-year-old is actually in better condition than a college student who has an average fitness level.

If you achieve a high level of fitness now and maintain it throughout your life, it will have a profound impact on the quality and quantity of your years. So, if you don't already exercise, start today.

## EXERCISE IMPROVES THE ABILITY TO FIGHT DISEASE

We explained in the previous chapter how exercise helps prevent all of the mostly deadly diseases. But not only does exercise reduce your risk of getting those diseases, it also improves the outcome if you do develop disease.

For example, years ago it was widely believed that exercise was dangerous after a heart attack or heart failure. This myth has been debunked. In fact, multiple analyses have concluded that regular exercise reduces mortality rates after a heart attack.

One noteworthy study looked at patients who were enrolled in an exercise program after having a coronary angioplasty, a method of opening a narrowed or blocked artery in the heart by inflating a small balloon inside the artery. The study showed that individuals on an exercise program had substantial improvement in exercise capacity and quality of life, fewer subsequent cardiac events, and one-third fewer hospital admissions than their sedentary counterparts.

Another study compared the benefits of exercise in younger people with coronary artery disease to the benefits of exercise in older people with heart disease. The people who were seventy years old or more showed improvements in exercise capacity, lipid levels, and body mass similar to those experienced by the patients in their early fifties. A recent study in the British journal *Heart* showed that becoming very active in late adulthood cuts coronary artery disease by 90 percent! So, no matter the age, prevention practices work and should be practiced—even among the elderly.

Exercise can be an effective treatment for patients with blockages in the arteries in their legs, known as peripheral artery disease. An analysis of twenty-one studies showed that, overall, an exercise program helped individuals increase by 179 percent the distance they walked pain-free. The greatest improvements in walking ability occurred when exercise lasted more than thirty minutes and took place at least three times per week for six months or more. And with walking there are no prescriptions to fill or co-pays to worry about!

## FIT AND FAT OR LEAN AND SEDENTARY— WHICH IS BETTER?

Is it more important to be fit or lean? Who is healthier, the fit, overweight person or the lean, sedentary one? Many studies have investigated this question, and the results suggest that exercise and fitness are more important than body weight. The Cooper Institute, using data from the Aerobics Center Longitudinal Study, has shown that increased fitness is associated with reduced mortality in all weight categories—normal, overweight, and obese. According to this study, the fitter you are, the lower your risk of mortality, no matter what you weigh.

However, we think both factors are important to control, and we recommend that you exercise often and keep your weight in the normal range. An important point to remember is that just because you may be lean, it doesn't mean that you don't need to get regular exercise. A study published in 2005 in the *Archives of Internal Medicine*

---

## Ways to "Sneak in" Exercise throughout the Day

Take the stairs, not the elevator
Park your car in the farthest location from your destination
Take an exercise break at work instead of a coffee break
Plan active vacations rather than driving trips
Spend time playing with your kids

---

found that diabetic men who were thin but out of shape had almost a three-fold higher rate of cardiovascular disease than those diabetic men who were overweight but in good physical shape. We all need regular exercise no matter what our weight.

Being fit is particularly important when you already have a disease and/or significant risk factors. Fit individuals with any combination of smoking, elevated blood pressure, and high cholesterol have lower death rates than sedentary individuals with *none* of these characteristics.

## WHAT ABOUT THE RISKS OF PHYSICAL ACTIVITY?

Study after study shows that the benefits of exercise far outweigh any harm caused by exercise. In fact, physical activity generally decreases injury risk and is recommended to reduce the incidence of falls in older adults.

Risk for injury does increase with obesity, the duration of exercise, and the intensity of the activity. The most common injuries from exercise occur in the muscles and bones, as well as the cartilage, ligaments, and tendons.

The general principle for reducing injury risk is to start exercising slowly, follow a carefully calibrated routine, and gradually increase exertion over time. If you are more than fifty years old, overweight, or have multiple cardiac risk factors, you should talk to your physician and get screened with a treadmill stress test before starting an exercise routine.

## GETTING STARTED AND STICKING WITH AN EXERCISE PROGRAM

The two hardest things about exercise are getting started and keeping with it.

You now know the enormous value of exercise, which should help motivate you to get started. Below are several of our suggestions for improving your chances of doing it correctly and sticking with your program.

Start slowly and don't overdo it. If you create goals that are too ambitious, you'll end up discouraged when you don't achieve them. And if you work out too hard too soon, you'll become exhausted and less likely to keep it up.

Instead, set short-term, achievable goals, such as, "Today I'm going to walk around the block." Do that for several days, until you get comfortable with it and gain confidence that you can stick to your goal. Then, when you're ready, make a new goal—consider increasing your walk to two, three, or four blocks, or maybe even a mile. Walk slowly at first, then faster and faster, swinging your arms. Eventually you may even get to a slow jog . . . then a run. You can do it once you set your mind to it!

Many people quit their exercise program because they don't give it a chance to become a habit. Research indicates that it takes about twenty-one days to establish a habit in your life. Set a goal to start a program and continue with it for a month. Once you've been doing an exercise routine for a month, you are much more likely to keep going.

Plan exercise into your day. This is your time to take care of yourself so you can enjoy a longer and healthier life. At night, when you are preparing for bed, plan your exercise and make sure everything you need is ready (equipment, gym bag, shoes, etc.).

Try to exercise at the same time every day—but be flexible and make sure you fit in some exercise even if you miss your designated time. Mornings are great for exercising, as there are typically fewer interruptions to derail your program. Plus, you will achieve your goals first thing in the morning and reap the benefits of exercise all day long, which will make you more likely to do it again the following day. Make exercise a priority; stick with your schedule.

Don't make excuses! Exercise even when you think you're "too tired." Exercise will actually give you energy, so you won't feel as tired.

Other ideas to help you stick with your exercise program:

**Exercise with a partner and surround yourself with supportive people**. This can make it a more enjoyable experience. Plus, you are accountable to someone other than yourself. Supportive people can help you stick with your goals.

**Make it fun.** Play music, vary your routine, try a new exercise, do the type of exercise you enjoy.

**Log your activity with a pedometer or in a journal**. This record will help you keep track of your exercise, meet your goals, and create new goals based on previous workouts.

**Don't get discouraged**. You may have a bad day or feel as if you're not making progress, but you are.

**Reward yourself.** After you've successfully fulfilled your goal to exercise for a month, treat yourself to new running shoes or a new workout outfit.

## WHAT TYPE OF EXERCISE IS BEST?

We recommend that your exercise regime include moderate physical activity, or something that will cause you to sweat and your heart to pump harder. This includes taking a brisk walk, riding a bike, swimming laps, or using cardiovascular equipment at the gym. The important thing is to do something that you like and stick with it.

If you're just starting out, walking is the best exercise. It's easy, cheap, and you can do it anywhere. All you need is a good pair of walking or running shoes and comfortable clothing. If it's too cold to walk outside, find a mall where you can walk before the stores open.

How important are strength training and stretching? Stretching and strength training are great ways to round out a good exercise plan. Strength training is beneficial to your bones and muscles, and it can help prevent osteoporosis. It improves strength, endurance, balance, and coordination. Stretching is also helpful. It improves flexibility and is great for warming up or cooling down from physical activity.

## HOW MUCH IS ENOUGH?

The U.S. Centers for Disease Control and Prevention, the American College of Sports Medicine, and the American Cancer Society recommend that every adult should accumulate thirty minutes or more of moderate-intensity physical activity on most, preferably all, days of the week. As little as thirty minutes of walking a day—which can even be split up into intervals (for example, ten minutes at a time)—will dramatically decrease your risk of developing many major causes of death in the United States, including heart disease and cancer.

## "I Thought I Was Bulletproof"

That was what Rob Umbreit, one of my friends, and a patient, said after suffering a heart attack while having surgery for prostate cancer. He was extremely fit, a helicopter skier and a competitive cyclist. He thought that a heart attack would never happen to him. But it did.

Exercise does not make you "immortal." You need to realize that there are many other components to a healthy life. This is one point that we make certain our fit, very athletic patients understand—exercise is only one of our 10 tips for longevity. —*Richard J. Flanigan, MD*

While thirty minutes of walking a day can improve your longevity, more activity will have an even greater effect. In an article published in the *American Journal of Epidemiology* in 1978, Dr. Ralph Paffenbarger showed that the biggest reduction in cardiovascular risk occurs at an exercise level that burns two thousand to three thousand calories per week. For a brisk walker, two thousand calories per week equates to approximately twenty miles (100 calories per mile). This averages out to just over three miles a day. In fact, exercise at levels that burn greater than three thousand calories per week causes some health risks to rise, mostly because of dehydration, electrolyte imbalance, and metabolic problems.

### EXERCISE RX: JUST DO IT!

Inertia, boredom, lack of time, bad memories of past gym classes. There are endless reasons why people stay sedentary when they know they should be moving. Exercise benefits your mind, your body, and your biochemistry in powerful ways. It's time now to make the commitment to exercise. Vigorous exercise is good, but even thirty minutes of brisk walking every day of the week can put you on track to achieve the ultimate goal: a long and healthy life.

## CHAPTER 5

# Diet: Personal Choices with Huge Impacts

"For the two out of three adult Americans who do not smoke and do not drink excessively, one personal choice seems to influence long-term health prospects more than any other: what we eat." So wrote Dr. C. Everett Koop in his 1988 *Surgeon General's Report on Nutrition and Health*. As he pointed out, overeating and dietary imbalances have been associated with coronary artery disease, stroke, diabetes, and cancer, which account for almost two-thirds of all deaths in the United States. In addition, he wrote, high blood pressure, obesity, dental disease, osteoporosis, and gastrointestinal diseases all result, at least in part, from poor diets.

Clearly, we must evaluate our own diets and make the proper choices in order to live long and healthy lives. A good place to start would be to learn about the diets of long-lived people.

## HEALTHY DIETS AROUND THE WORLD

In November 2005, *National Geographic* magazine published a fascinating article entitled "The Secrets of Long Life," by Dan Buettner. Buettner's article looked at some of the longest-lived populations in the world: the Okinawans in Japan, the Sardinians in Italy, and the Seventh-day Adventists in Loma Linda, California. Buettner found that each of these three groups shared a number of fundamental habits: being physically active; being less stressed; and eating diets rich in fruits, vegetables, and whole grains.

So what else can we learn from these groups? Let's first take a look at the Japanese, Mediterranean, and vegetarian diets to see what we can uncover about increasing the quality and quantity of our lives.

### Japanese diet: Fish, legumes, and hara hachi bu

Japanese people eat fifty times more fish than Americans do. We Americans eat thirty-five times more meat than the Japanese. Japanese eat ninety times more legumes—beans, peas, peanuts, lentils, soybeans, and soy products—than Americans do. The soy intake on the Japanese island of Okinawa is 100 grams a day. In the United States it is 1. The Okinawans consume an average of 1,800 calories a day. Americans consume an average of 2,500 calories a day.

The Okinawans understand that your body is a bit slow to let your brain know when your appetite has been satisfied. They know that your brain will catch up with the message from your stomach in fifteen to twenty minutes. Hence, they subscribe to the Confucian-based dictum *"hara hachi bu,"* which means eat until you feel 80 percent full. Otherwise, if you eat until you are 100 percent full, you will overeat by approximately 20 percent.

**U.S., Mediterranean, and Japanese Diets Compared**

|                             | *United States* | *Crete/Corfu* | *Japan* |
| --------------------------- | --------------- | ------------- | ------- |
| Percentage fat              | 39              | 37            | 11      |
| Percentage saturated fat    | 18              | 8             | 3       |
| Legumes (grams/day)         | 1               | 30            | 91      |
| Breads/cereals (grams/day)  | 123             | 453           | 481     |
| Meat (grams/day)            | 273             | 35            | 8       |
| Fish (grams/day)            | 3               | 39            | 150     |

*Source:* Reprinted with the permission of Simon & Schuster Adult Publishing Group from *Eat, Drink, and Be Healthy* by Walter C. Willett, MD, © 2001 and 2005 by President and Fellows of Harvard College.

### Mediterranean diet: Monounsaturated fats

Now take a look at the Mediterranean diet. It is probably the best diet in the world, with the lowest incidence of heart disease. What may surprise you is that the intake of fat in Mediterranean countries, such as Italy, Greece, and Spain, is higher than it is in Finland, which has some of the highest rates of heart disease and saturated fat consumption in the world. The difference between the two populations is the type of fat consumed. The Mediterranean diet uses almost all monounsaturated fats, which are found in olive oil, canola oil, nuts, and avocados. In Finland, the main type of fat consumed is saturated fat, found in dairy products and red meat.

### Vegetarian diet: Fruits, vegetables, and no meat

By definition, a vegetarian diet is rich in fruits and vegetables, and excludes meat, which often has high levels of saturated fat and cholesterol. Vegetarian diets can significantly reduce one's risk of contracting heart disease, colon and lung cancer, osteoporosis, diabetes, kidney disease, hypertension, obesity, and a number of other debilitating conditions. The Seventh-day Adventists in Loma Linda are a testament to this.

The National Institutes of Health funded a twelve-year study of thirty-four thousand Adventists to determine whether their lifestyle and vegetarian diets affected their life expectancy and risk of disease. The researchers concluded that not only did the Adventists' diet lower the risks of developing certain cancers and heart disease, but it also added up to ten years to their average life span.

With that in mind, we recommend eating several vegetarian meals each week, even if you are not a vegetarian. But don't substitute the red meat for another high-saturated-fat product such as cheese. Be creative. You'll be surprised how satisfying vegetarian meals can be.

Just a quick note on veganism, which is a way of life and not just a diet. Vegans do not eat meat or eggs, they do not drink milk, and often they don't eat sugar or honey. Adherent vegans don't use leather, silk, or down products.

There is no question that a vegan diet can be healthy, but it can also make it challenging to get the essential vitamins, minerals, and protein your body requires. And this strict diet can be very difficult to follow. Vegans and vegetarians also miss out on the great health benefits of eating fish.

Instead, we recommend that you focus on our list of "superfoods" and exercise regularly. (For superfoods list, see page 76.) In doing so, your health benefits can be great, your life span increased, and your adherence to a healthy diet much easier to maintain.

What essential lessons do the Mediterranean, Japanese, and vegetarian diets offer? Eat less meat and more fish, legumes, and monounsaturated fats. And eat only until you are 80 percent full. *Hara hachi bu!*

## Fat: Explaining the Differences

There are four main types of fat: saturated, monounsaturated, polyunsaturated, and trans fat.

Monounsaturated fat and polyunsaturated fat are "good" fats that are heart-healthy and actually lower cholesterol. Polyunsaturated fats come from plant oils such as safflower, sesame, soy, corn, and sunflower-seed oils, as well as nuts and seeds. Fish oils are polyunsaturated fats that contain the health-promoting omega-3 fatty acids. Monounsaturated fats also come from plant oils, such as those found in olives, rapeseeds (source of canola oil), peanuts, and avocados.

Saturated and trans fats are the "bad" fats. They increase our bad cholesterol and lower our good cholesterol, leading to heart disease. They also contribute to the hardening and clogging of our arteries. Saturated fats are found in animal meats, dairy products, such as whole milk and cheese, and some plant sources, such as palm oil and cocoa butter.

The American Heart Association recommends that you limit saturated fat consumption to about fifteen to nineteen grams per day, which amounts to a little more than two tablespoons of butter.

Trans fats are even worse for you than saturated fats. While trans fats naturally occur in small amounts, the vast majority of trans fats that people consume are artificial. Trans fats are created during the process of partial hydrogenation of vegetable oils. This is a process that has been used for decades to make oil more solid (like shortening) by adding hydrogen atoms to the fat molecules.

Hydrogenation provides longer shelf-life in baked products and longer fry-life for cooking oils. Some believe it improves the texture and taste of processed foods. Trans fats are found primarily in baked goods, such as cookies, crackers, cakes, and donuts, as well as in deep-fried foods, such as French fries and fried onion rings.

The American Heart Association (AHA) recommends that your daily intake of trans fats be limited to 1 percent of total calories, which is equivalent to roughly two to two-and-a-half grams of trans fat per day. It is important to know that trans fats are found in foods that carry the label "partially hydrogenated."

## Rising Tide against Trans Fats

Opponents of trans fats are becoming widespread and have surprisingly political and powerful voices in America. Take a look at the informative Web site Ban Trans Fats (www.bantransfats.com). This is the group that sued Kraft Foods for providing artery-clogging trans fats to our children in the form of Oreo cookies. And they won.

The publicity surrounding that lawsuit created huge public awareness about the trans fat issue. It also triggered an avalanche of events, including the U.S. Food and Drug Administration (FDA) rule, effective January 1, 2006, that requires all packaged foods to list trans fat content on their labels.

Major fast food chains are joining the ban on trans fats. KFC announced in October 2006 that its restaurants were switching to trans fat–free oils. Wendy's and McDonald's have announced plans to cut trans fats.

On December 5, 2006, New York City passed an initiative requiring all restaurants to stop using cooking oils, shortening, and spreads that contain more than 0.5 grams of trans fat per serving by July 2007, and to stop serving any foods containing trans fats by July 2008.

Walter Willett, MD, professor of Epidemiology and Nutrition at the Harvard School of Public Health, said, "If New Yorkers replace all sources of artificial trans fat, by even the most conservative estimates, at least five hundred deaths from heart disease would be prevented each year in New York City—more than the number of people killed annually in motor vehicle crashes. Based on long-term studies, the number of preventable deaths may be many times higher. Trans fat from partially hydrogenated vegetable oil is a toxic substance that does not belong in food."

## "SUPERFOODS": WHAT ARE THE BEST FOODS TO EAT?

Our patients often ask us which foods are the most nutritious. The Mayo Clinic lists ten "Best Bets" on its Web site: apples, almonds, blueberries, broccoli, red beans, salmon, spinach, sweet potatoes, vegetable juice, and wheat germ.

In January 2002, the editors at *Time* magazine published their list of "Ten Foods That Pack a Wallop." They agreed that broccoli, salmon, spinach, blueberries, and nuts are excellent foods, but also included tomatoes, red wine, oats, garlic, and green tea. In December 2003, *Nutrition Action Healthletter*, which publishes one of the best health-promoting newsletters in this country, listed its top ten superfoods: sweet potatoes, grape tomatoes, fat-free or 1 percent milk, broccoli, salmon, whole grain crackers, brown rice, citrus fruits, butternut squash, and greens, including kale and spinach.

We have looked extensively at the published nutritional literature and have found even more foods to add to these compelling lists. In addition to the items mentioned above, there are plenty of data to support avocados, olive oil, bell peppers, cruciferous vegetables (broccoli and Brussels sprouts), legumes, and plant stanols and sterols. (See sidebar "What Are Plant Stanols and Sterols?" on page 78.) Take a look at the *Longevity Made Simple* list of superfoods, which appears on the next page. It contains twenty-two of our favorite nutritious foods, each scientifically proven to deliver powerful health benefits.

We recommend incorporating as many of these twenty-two foods as you can into your diet. These foods, along with exercise, offer some of the best protection available against developing a variety of diseases and will contribute greatly to your longevity.

## *LONGEVITY MADE SIMPLE* LIST OF "SUPERFOODS"

**Almonds and walnuts** (and other nuts)—Lower both total and LDL cholesterol levels.

**Apples**—Low in calories, high in soluble fiber, which helps lower cholesterol.

**Avocados**—Rich in monounsaturated fat and fiber; source of plant sterol and antioxidants.

**Bell peppers**—Great source of beta-carotene and vitamin C; rich in bioflavonoids and phenols.

**Blueberries** (and other berries)—Great source of antioxidants and dietary fiber.

**Citrus fruits**—Lots of vitamin C, folate, thiamine, and potassium.

**Cruciferous vegetables**—Have unique compounds that are felt to be cancer protective. Specifically, they contain a sulfur-containing compound that gives them the pungent taste that we notice in Brussels sprouts, broccoli, cauliflower, cabbage, and bok choy.

**Fat-free or 1 percent milk** (and yogurt)—Excellent source of calcium.

**Garlic** (and onions)—Linked to anticlotting, cholesterol lowering, and cancer protection.

**Legumes** (including beans, peas, lentils, peanuts, and soy)—Vegetarian source of protein, low in calories and saturated fat, good source of vitamin B6, potassium, and zinc.

**Melons**—Good source of lycopene and vitamin C.

**Olive oil** (particularly virgin olive oil)—Beneficial to your health not only for its monounsaturated fat (oleic acid), but also because it is rich in polyphenols. Polyphenol intake has been associated with low cancer and coronary artery disease mortality rates—likely due to antioxidant and anti-inflammatory properties. Virgin olive oil has higher phenolic content than regular olive oil.

**Plant stanols and sterols**—Reduce absorption of dietary cholesterol in the intestines, thus lowering cholesterol levels in blood.

**Red wine**—Contains bioflavonoids, phenols, resveratrol, and tannins, which have antioxidant and anticlotting properties; raises HDL cholesterol.

**Salmon** (and other fish)—Rich in omega-3 fatty acids; great source of protein and iron.

**Spinach**—Source of vitamins A, K, C, and B6; riboflavin; folate; and potassium.

**Squash**—Great source of beta-carotene, potassium, fiber, folate, and vitamins A and C.

**Sweet potatoes**—High in fiber, beta-carotene, vitamins C and B6, folate, and potassium.

**Tea** (green or black)—Contains antioxidants, bioflavonoids, and tannins.

**Tomatoes**—Rich in lycopene, an antioxidant that protects against some cancers; good source of vitamin C, folate, and potassium.

**Vegetable juice**—Great way to include vegetables in your diet; contains many vitamins, minerals, and other nutrients; choose reduced-sodium juice or, better yet, make your own juice in a blender with whole vegetables.

**Whole grains** (including brown rice, oats, wheat germ, and whole wheat)—Good source of vitamin E, zinc, thiamine, folate, magnesium, and fiber.

Healthy foods not only lower your weight and cholesterol levels and provide the essential vitamins, minerals, and nutrients you need on a daily basis, but they also work at a biochemical level to reduce oxidative stress, reduce inflammation, improve the elasticity of your arteries, improve insulin sensitivity, improve blood pressure, and decrease clotting tendencies. This is important because these mechanisms have been found to play a role in preventing heart disease, stroke, cancer, and diabetes.

## What Are Plant Stanols and Sterols?

Plant stanols and sterols have a chemical makeup similar to cholesterol. Foods enriched with plant stanols or sterols lower serum cholesterol levels by reducing the body's absorption of cholesterol. By doing so, they have been found to lower LDL cholesterol levels. Research has shown that the intake of two grams per day of stanols or sterols reduced low-density lipoprotein (LDL) by 10 percent. And if you are watching your diet by eating foods low in saturated fat and cholesterol and high in stanols or sterols, you can reduce LDL cholesterol by 20 percent. Furthermore, adding sterol or stanol to your diet while taking a statin medication is more effective than doubling the statin dose! Long-term use of stanols and/or sterols is likely to lower the risk of coronary artery disease by 12 percent to 20 percent in the first five years, and by 20 percent over a lifetime. At this time, the best sources of stanols and sterols are orange juice and butter spreads such as Benecol and Take Control. These spreads are good for you, so don't be afraid to slather them on your whole-wheat toast.

## FOODS THAT HARM

On the other hand, it is important to note that there are also harmful foods that actually promote disease. These unhealthy foods contribute to oxidative stress, inflammation, decreased arterial elasticity, decreased insulin sensitivity, elevated blood pressure, and greater clotting tendencies. We have already discussed the need to limit your intake of saturated and trans fats found in red meat, fried foods, and processed baked goods. Strictly limit your consumption of processed meats, such as hot dogs, sausage, scrapple, and bacon. You should also avoid or limit your intake of refined starches and sugars, such as those found in white bread, soda, and candy bars. These foods are highly processed, resulting in the removal of fiber, vitamins, minerals, phytonutrients, and essential fatty acids.

## A FISH TALE: HOW TO GET YOUR OMEGA-3 FATTY ACIDS

The powerful nutritional benefit of fish lies in the fact that it contains a high amount of omega-3 fatty acids. We need omega-3 fatty acids for the normal functioning of our bodies—they are used in cell membranes throughout the body; they are building blocks for hormones; they have a role in regulating blood clotting; they minimize inflammation; and they improve arterial elasticity. They also help keep your heart beating normally by regulating your heart's rhythm.

Omega-3 fatty acids are obtained from two dietary sources: seafood and plant oils. Fish and fish oils contain the most potent omega-3 fatty acids, EPA (eicosapentaenoic acid) and DHA (docosahexaenoic acid). The plant oils found in canola oil, soybeans (tofu), flaxseed, and nuts (particularly walnuts) contain the less potent omega-3 fatty acid, ALA (alpha-linolenic acid).

The evidence is overwhelming that these fatty acids are beneficial for your heart. For example, one extensive thirty-

### Benefits of Omega-3 Fatty Acids

Reduce inflammation
Help prevent the formation of
  blood clots
Help correct irregular heartbeats
Reduce coronary artery disease
Help prevent heart attacks
Help prevent strokes
Reduce all-cause mortality
Lower triglycerides
Stabilize plaques
Improve endothelial function

*Source:* Jennifer G. Robinson, MD, MPH, and Neil J. Stone, MD, "Antiatherosclerotic and Antithrombotic Effects of Omega-3 Fatty Acids," *The American Journal of Cardiology,* August 21, 2006.

**How to Get Your Omega-3 Fatty Acids from Fish**

| Fish | Grams of omega-3 fatty acids in a 100-gram (3.5-ounce) serving of fish |
| --- | --- |
| Herring | 2.1–2.2 |
| Salmon | 1.8–2.3 (lox—0.5) |
| Sardines (canned) | 1.5–1.6 |
| Mackerel | 1.3–1.9 (king mackerel—0.4) |
| Trout | 1.1–1.2 |
| Halibut | 0.5–1.2 (Greenland halibut high) |
| Tuna (fresh) | 0.3–1.5 (bluefin high; skipjack, yellowfin low) |
| Shrimp (canned) | 0.6 |
| Flounder/Sole | 0.5 |
| Crab | 0.4–0.5 |
| Scallops | 0.4 |
| Shrimp (fresh) | 0.3 |
| Catfish | 0.3–0.5 |
| Tuna (canned) | 0.2–0.4 |
| Cod | 0.2–0.3 |
| Lobster (northern) | 0.1 |

*Source:* USDA National Nutrient Database for Standard Reference, Release 19 (2006), Finfish and Shellfish Products.

year study showed that men who consumed two servings of fish a week had a 38 percent lower risk of heart attack than men who did not eat fish. The men who ate fish also had a 67 percent reduced risk of sudden death from heart attack.

There is also a clear dose-response relationship—that is, the more you eat, the better the effect. In the Nurses' Health Study, researchers demonstrated a significant reduction in death from coronary artery disease with increasing intake of omega-3 fatty acids. Women who ate fish at least five times a week had a 34 percent lower risk of death from coronary artery disease than those women who consumed fish less than once a month. In a large physicians' health study, the risk of sudden death was 81 percent less in those people who ate the most fish, compared to those who ate none. Even among those who consumed low to moderate amounts of fish, the risk of sudden death was 52 percent lower than those who consumed fish less than once a month.

Two important studies demonstrated the benefits of fish in reducing deaths from stroke, in both men and women, young and old, with varying amounts of fish consumed. In fact, one of these studies even suggested that consumption of at least one portion of fish a week may be associated with lower stroke rates. The other study showed that consumption of fish is associated with lower risk of stroke among elderly.

Another interesting piece of data, published in the July 2003 *Archives of Neurology*, showed a connection between fish and Alzheimer's disease. The study noted that one or more servings of fish per week resulted in a 60 percent reduced risk of Alzheimer's disease. Johanna M. Seddon, MD, also reported that regular consumption of fish reduced the risk of macular degeneration, a devastating vision problem common in the elderly, by 45 percent.

### How much to eat

In order to get the recommended amount of omega-3 fatty acids, the American Heart Association recommends that all adults eat fish (which is also a good source of protein and low in saturated fat) at least two times a week. The "fatty" fish, particularly salmon, sardines, mackerel, herring, tuna, and trout, have significant amounts of cardioprotective omega-3 fatty acids. Farm-raised salmon and trout contain similar amounts of omega-3 fatty acids as their wild counterparts. Many fried fish, however, have been shown to have no benefit and, in fact, are unhealthy. They are low in omega-3 fatty acids and high in trans fats.

For individuals with documented heart disease, the American Heart Association recommends one gram of EPA and DHA per day.

## Precautions about Fish

Sometimes fish contain significant levels of methylmercury, polychlorinated biphenyls (PCB), dioxins and other environmental contaminants. Most of these are generally found in older, larger predatory fish, such as shark, swordfish, mackerel, and tilefish. Fish with the lowest levels of mercury include salmon (wild and farmed), oysters, clams, haddock, shrimp, and flounder/sole.

The dangers of methylmercury generally depend on the level of exposure. It is known that very high mercury exposures following industrial or occupational accidents can cause health effects that include problems with the nervous system. Health effects from low-level exposure, such as that seen from fish consumption, are less understood. Although this issue needs to be further studied, it is clearly understood that eating a variety of different fish will decrease the likelihood of excess mercury or PCB exposure.

Having reviewed the scientific data on contaminants such as PCB and mercury, as well as the data on the health benefits of one to two servings of fish a week, we have concluded that for middle-aged and older men and women, the benefits of eating fish far outweigh the rare risks of mercury toxicity.

It is important to mention that children and pregnant or nursing women are at highest risk for potential problems associated with exposure to excessive mercury. According to the FDA, these individuals should avoid fish high in mercury (shark, swordfish, mackerel, and tilefish).

The FDA provides information on mercury levels in different fish on its Web site, www.cfsan.fda.gov/seafood1.html.

Most fish and fish oil pills have both EPA and DHA. In some patients with very high triglycerides (for example, 500 mg/dL), three to four grams of EPA and DHA are recommended per day. This can lower triglycerides by 20 to 40 percent. However, taking this high amount of fish oil can increase bleeding tendencies, so take these quantities only under the care of a physician.

If you do not particularly like fish, eat as much as you can tolerate and supplement it with fish oil capsules—one a day, or up to two or three a day, depending on your risk of heart disease. Not all capsules contain the same amount of omega-3 fatty acids—make sure you look closely at the label and talk to your physician about the proper dosage.

## NUTS

There have been more than thirty scientific studies showing that nuts can significantly reduce the risk of heart disease. One study in 1992 showed that Seventh-day Adventists who ate nuts at least four times a week suffered 51 percent fewer heart attacks than those who ate less. The Nurses' Health Study found that women who ate five or more ounces of nuts per week reduced their risk of heart disease by 35 percent. The Physicians' Health Study showed that participants who ate nuts at least twice a week had half the rate of sudden death as those who rarely or never ate nuts.

Nuts (including nut butters and nut oils) have been found to lower total cholesterol between 2 percent and 16 percent and LDL cholesterol between 2 percent and 19 percent, when compared to people not consuming nuts. Most physicians who ate nuts at least twice a week had half the rate of sudden cardiac death than those who rarely or never ate nuts.

Remember, however, that nuts do have a large amount of fat and calories. The fat is mostly unsaturated, which is heart-healthy. But calories do count. So just like everything else, consume them in moderation. Eat about an ounce a day, which is approximately one handful. Some people recommend eating your nuts from a shell, which takes a little longer and will help you eat less.

## Which Nuts Are Best?

Not all nuts are equal. When the FDA approved a health claim for nuts on food labels, it applied to the following types of nuts:

walnuts

almonds

pine nuts

pecans

pistachios

hazelnuts

peanuts—They are not truly a nut but are classified as a legume. Peanut butter is often supplemented with hydrogenated fat, which takes away the health benefits. If you want to enjoy the benefits of peanuts, choose the natural, unhydrogenated peanut butter (oil rises to the top).

The FDA did not allow health claims for macadamia nuts, Brazil nuts, and cashews because they contain too much saturated fat.

Thanks to the fat content, however, nuts do make us feel full and satisfied. Studies have shown that those who regularly ate nuts weighed less than those who did not.

## TEA: AS CLOSE AS YOU CAN GET TO A MAGIC POTION

Whether it's green or black, tea has powerful qualities that can help prevent cancer and cardiovascular disease. In fact, tea may be one of the best health drinks ever.

Researchers have been touting the benefits of tea for several years. Both black and green teas contain polyphenols, powerful antioxidants that make it a magic potion. Antioxidants neutralize damaging effects of free radicals present in the body. Free radicals are made of unstable oxygen molecules that react with and damage our cells, which can lead to cancer and cardiovascular disease.

Herbal teas have not been shown to provide these beneficial effects, as they do not contain polyphenols.

The more processed the leaf, the darker it will become. Green tea is the least processed tea and contains the most antioxidants. Black tea is partially dried, crushed, and fermented. This process destroys about 10 percent of its powerful antioxidant qualities. Whether black or green, hot or iced, two cups of tea a day is what we recommend.

## WHAT ABOUT COFFEE?

More Americans drink coffee rather than drink tea. It had been previously thought that coffee was unhealthy, but much of that was due to coffee drinkers who also smoked cigarettes and, thus, had a greater incidence of cancer. It was the cigarettes that made coffee look bad. Recent studies have been able to separate cigarettes as a factor, and they have not been able to show detrimental health effects due to coffee drinking alone.

Recent studies have actually shown that coffee has a high level of antioxidants and, therefore, is quite healthy. In fact, one study in postmenopausal women showed that consumption of coffee is associated with reduced inflammation, which may reduce the risk of cardiovascular disease and other inflammatory diseases. Coffee consumption has also been associated with a lower risk for diabetes in both men and women. We recommend drinking no more than four eight-ounce cups of coffee a day.

So you are getting some health benefits whether you choose to drink coffee or tea.

## EAT LESS, BUT FEEL LIKE YOU ARE EATING MORE

Restricted calorie diets have been touted in the news for the past few years as the key to longevity. Recent studies have shown that mice that consumed about 25 percent fewer calories than mice on a regular diet live about 25 percent longer. Several researchers, including Roy and Lisa Walford, believe that the benefits of restricted-calorie diets will benefit humans as well. We agree with these authors, and we believe that calorie restriction is a way to lose weight and to improve longevity.

The only problem is the feasibility of such a diet. It would be very difficult for most people to significantly restrict their caloric intake in our "supersize me" society. Deprivation doesn't feel very good, and it sometimes results in the opposite effect—overeating.

We recommend that you choose an approach that is more likely to work for you, one that will help you eat less, but not feel deprived. You can eat a variety of foods that make you feel full and satisfied but don't overload you with calories.

Satiety is the key to weight control. Your gastrointestinal system sends satiety signals to your brain telling it that you are full. These signals are stretching of the stomach, hormones, and insulin. When food fills your stomach, it stretches and releases satiety signals to your brain. As your stomach fills, satiety hormones are also released. And as food is digested, some of its calories are converted into blood glucose, which causes insulin levels to rise and provides another signal to the brain that the body is being fed.

But you need to give your brain time to process the signals. It takes about fifteen to twenty minutes before the brain registers that you are eating and turns off the hunger signals. So, eat slowly and remember the Okinawans' 80 percent rule, *hara hachi bu.* (See page 70.)

We are impressed and inspired by the writings of Barbara Rolls from Pennsylvania State University. She coined the term "volumetrics" and has written several books regarding this concept and its impact on weight control. Dr. Rolls's strategy for weight control is to eat a satisfying volume of food while controlling calories and meeting nutrient requirements.

Dr. Rolls points out that foods with high water content have a big impact on satiety. Water, by itself, quenches thirst but does not abate hunger. Water in food, however, contributes to satiety; it adds volume without contributing calories. Foods that have higher water content include fruits, vegetables, low-fat milk, cut greens, lean meats, poultry, fish, and beans. Water-rich dishes, such as soups, stews, casseroles, pasta with vegetables, and fruit-based desserts, will increase the volume of food in your stomach and suppress your appetite sooner than foods lower in water content.

## Soup

That's why we like soup. Eating soup at the beginning of a meal is a fabulous way to abate hunger. It has a large volume and high water content, which increase satiety without increasing calories. Hot soup also helps with the satiety signals because you cannot gulp it down quickly. Sipping it slowly helps pass the twenty minutes that it takes for your brain to get the signal that it is full. Then, when it's time for the rest of the meal, the signals of satiety are starting to register, and you will be less inclined to eat too much.

Dr. Rolls discussed a study in her book, *The Volumetrics Weight-Control Plan,* that found that the more soup people ate, the fewer calories they took in and the more weight they lost. So, take your time while eating and consider having a nice, hot bowl of soup to start your next meal, or better yet, as your whole meal.

## PLAN AHEAD AND LISTEN TO YOUR BODY

It is essential that you develop a healthy eating plan that you know you can follow, regardless of whether it's a specific diet.

Plan ahead. Know what you are going to eat each day and ensure that you have that food available to make it happen. If you prepare your menu on the spur of the moment, you will be more likely to choose something easy—fast food or a frozen pizza or even a carton of ice cream—rather than a healthy, nutritious meal.

Another good tip from Barbara Rolls is to ask yourself, "Am I hungry?" at the beginning of a meal and rate your hunger on a scale from one to ten. As you eat, pause periodically and ask yourself again, "Am I still hungry?" Once your rating has reached a five, it is a good time to stop eating.

## DON'T FORGET THE SNACKS

Hunger can be more easily satisfied than many people realize. In addition to three meals a day, a snack in the mid-morning and one in the mid-afternoon of just 100 calories—an apple, a yogurt, or a handful of nuts—will suppress your appetite and get you through the entire day. The key to weight control is to eat often enough that you do not get very hungry. When you are famished, you are more likely to binge on anything that is at hand.

## PORTION CONTROL

Portion control is another key to healthy eating. We have to reprogram our thinking about what is a normal portion size. Imagine a deck of cards, your computer mouse, three dominos. A deck of cards should be the size of the steak that you eat, your computer mouse should be the amount of pasta that you have, and three dominoes should approximate the amount of cheese you consume. A burrito should be the size of a bar of soap. You know those burrito stores popping up all over the country? Are the burritos the size of a bar of soap? More like four bars of soap. In fact, the barbacoa burrito at Chipotle is gigantic—it has 1,300 calories! Do you really need to eat the whole thing? You know the answer: you don't!

It also may be helpful to use a smaller plate when serving food. The larger the plate size, the more food you can consume. The November 2006 *Nutrition Action Healthletter* described a study at Cornell University where researchers asked individuals to serve themselves ice cream. They were given large and small bowls and serving spoons. Those who received a larger bowl served and ate 31 percent more ice cream than those with the smaller bowl. And those with both the large spoon and large bowl ate 57 percent more ice cream than those with the small bowl and small spoon. The large bowl recipients did not realize they had served themselves more ice cream than the small bowl recipients. Using a smaller plate or bowl may be a great way to trick yourself into eating less!

Remember, plan ahead, choose super foods, control your portions, and *hara hachi bu.* Follow these recommendations, and you will be well on your way to a healthy diet. The American Dietetic Association says that eating 100 extra calories per day could add up to ten extra pounds per year on the waistline—don't let the pounds creep up on you. Changes don't have to be drastic; eating a little less each day will make a difference.

## CHAPTER 6

# Mental Health: Live Better, Live Longer

Thus far, we have focused on presenting the scientific evidence that can help you take better care of your body. But there is more to health and longevity than tending to your physical well-being. More than two thousand years ago, the Greek physician Hippocrates realized that your state of mind can influence your physical state of health. Today, there is a growing body of scientific evidence that bears out Hippocrates' original belief.

In this chapter we will describe research that shows how some personality traits, especially hostility and distress, can harm your health, and how to temper their negative effects. We will also discuss the negative impact of anxiety and depression and point out the value of seeking help for those problems. We will emphasize the importance of maintaining social connections to friends, family, and community, and of happiness in general. After reading this chapter, you will realize just how important your mental state of mind is to your physical well-being. And if you follow our recommendations, you will live not only a longer life, but a happier, more satisfying one as well.

## IS YOUR PERSONALITY AFFECTING YOUR HEALTH?

In the 1960s and 1970s, researchers first began to study the effects of personality on health. They categorized personalities into Type A, Type B, and Type C. The Type A behavior pattern was characterized by an excessive competitive drive, impatience, and anger/hostility. Type A personalities were thought to be prime candidates for heart disease. Type B personalities were considered the healthiest—relaxed and noncompetitive. And Type C personalities—outwardly pleasant people who avoid conflict by suppressing their feelings—were said to be cancer-prone. The theory pretty much fell apart in the late 1980s when large-scale studies found no reliable connection between the Type A personality and heart disease.

While the research did not support the theory that Type A behavior was connected to heart disease, it did demonstrate a link with one trait of the Type A personality, hostility. Hostile people, those with angry feelings, mistrustful attitudes, and aggressive behavior, had a 50 percent higher rate of coronary artery disease than those who rated low on the hostility scale.

In recent years, researchers have described a fourth personality type. Type D personality refers to a "distressed personality," which Belgian researcher Johan Denollet defines in terms of two emotional states: "negative affectivity" (worry, irritability, gloom) and "social inhibition" (being ill at ease around people and afraid to open up). People with distressed personalities are basically unhappy people who keep their negative emotions bottled up inside.

Dr. Denollet found that high distress scores are strongly associated with both hypertension and heart disease. Among individuals who already have heart disease, those with the highest distress scores are less responsive to treatment and have a poorer quality of life. In 1996, Dr. Denollet reported that cardiac patients with a Type D personality had death rates four times higher than other cardiac patients.

## MANAGING STRESS TO REDUCE OR PREVENT DISEASE

Personality traits such as anger, hostility, irritability, and gloominess increase the amount of stress we experience in our lives. But even easygoing Type B personalities are subject to the adverse physical effects of stress. Stressful situations can raise heart rate and blood pressure, which increases the heart's requirement for oxygen—and leads to chest pain in people who already have heart disease. During stressful times, our nervous system releases stress hormones such as adrenaline and cortisol. Adrenaline raises blood pressure and can contribute to an injury to the lining of your arteries, setting the stage for plaque buildup. Cortisol can suppress the immune system. Stress also increases the amount of blood-clotting factors that circulate in your blood. Once clots form, they can block an artery narrowed by plaque and lead to a heart attack.

Stress also has the tendency to affect our behavior. Have you ever found yourself overeating for comfort, smoking more, or exercising less when you're stressed?

So, what can you do about stress? The people in the New England Centenarian Study once again offer us insight into the factors that promote longevity. None of the 100-year-old people in the study lived free from stress and hardship. In fact, many had lived through very stressful times—the devastation of World War II, the loss of loved ones, and the Great Depression. Yet, they all managed to live more than a century. Thomas Perls, head of the study, believes that personality was the most important factor in their longevity. They had personalities that helped them deal with the stress "effectively and efficiently," thus protecting them from the physical and psychological damage that could have shortened their lives.

Many of us do not have personalities for dealing so well with stress. And it can be almost impossible to change your personality; it is who you are, and most scientists believe it is established early in life. But there are things you can do to reduce or to cope with stress. No matter what your personality type, we recommend that you incorporate stress-reduction techniques into your life. If you experience significant amounts of anger, hostility, and distress, it is even more important to reduce your stress levels and counter the negative effects of these personality traits.

Scientific research has linked stress-reduction techniques with improved health. For example, in 2004, researchers reported that meditation can lower blood pressure, thus reducing your risk of heart disease and stroke. In one set of results, African-American adolescents with high blood pressure who practiced transcendental meditation had greater decreases in blood pressure compared with individuals who did not practice meditation.

Another study looked at individuals who practiced yoga and meditation for an hour and a half, three times a week, for six weeks. Those practicing yoga and meditation significantly reduced their blood pressure, heart rate, and body mass index. Among people with coronary artery disease, yoga and meditation improved the responsiveness and flexibility of their arteries by 69 percent.

Whatever you choose for stress reduction—yoga, meditation, exercise, deep-breathing—try to make time for this every day, even if it is only for a few minutes.

## ANXIETY AND DEPRESSION

While some personality traits are next to immutable, other emotional and mental states are more amenable to change. Among these, anxiety and depression have been repeatedly linked to poorer health and shorter lives. In a study of 222 people who had experienced a heart attack, patients who were depressed in the week following the heart attack had more than six times the risk of dying in the next eighteen months compared with patients who were not depressed. A recent review of psychosocial factors and cardiovascular health found that anxiety and depression were associated with negative health impacts more than any other factors; eleven out of the eleven studies reviewed linked anxiety and depression to increased risk of heart attack, stroke, and/or death.

The good news is that anxiety and depression are both treatable conditions. In fact, the U.S. National Institute of Mental Health states that the treatment success rate for depression is 80 percent, better than the success rate for cardiovascular disease. Anxiety disorders can be successfully treated in 70 percent to 90 percent of the cases. So, if difficult times in your life are causing you to be depressed or anxious, don't just try to ride it out. Seek help. Talk to your doctor. Therapy and medications can help you feel better and, as a result, live healthier and longer.

## HAPPINESS HELPS US LIVE A LONGER, BETTER LIFE

If negative emotions such as hostility and distress can shorten our lives, can positive emotions lengthen them? There is support for the idea that having a positive outlook on life, being happy, leads to a longer life.

In one interesting study of nuns in Milwaukee, researchers examined the diaries of the sisters of Notre Dame at the time they joined the convent in the 1930s. They counted the number of times the nuns used positive and negative words, then used those counts to categorize each nun as having a more positive or less positive personality. These nuns went on to live almost the same life—they lived together, ate together, did mostly the same work. But when researchers looked at their longevity, they discovered, interestingly enough, that two-thirds of the less positive nuns died before their eighty-fifth birthday. Among the more positive nuns, 90 percent were still alive at age eighty-five. On average, the happiest nuns lived about nine years longer than the least happy nuns. Nine years is a pretty nice bonus for living a happy life.

Exactly how happiness helps us live longer is unclear, but it may be through a stronger immune system. One recent study looked at immune and endocrine factors in response to pleasant stimuli. The results showed that experiences that induced pleasant emotions increased blood levels of the disease-fighting molecule immunoglobulin A, and decreased levels of the stress hormone cortisol, which impairs the immune function.

## WHAT MAKES US HAPPY?

So, what makes us happy? Many factors have been identified, as we list on the next page. But one of the most strongly supported sources of happiness is your social network. People who have satisfying marriages, good friends, and participate in religious or community organizations are generally happier and more satisfied, and enjoy better health and longer lives.

Lisa Berkman, of the Harvard School of Public Health, and S. Leonard Syme, of the University of California at Berkeley, conducted a classic study of almost seven thousand adults in Alameda County, California, ranging in age from thirty-eight to ninety-four. Nine years after these people were first interviewed, men with the fewest social and community ties were 2.3 times as likely to have died as those with the most social and community ties. The most isolated women were 2.8 times more likely to die than their socially engaged counterparts. Those findings held up when the group was assessed again after seventeen years, as well as in a similar study conducted in Evans County, Georgia.

While personality is difficult to change, you can change your social network. Get involved, get outside of yourself, and connect with friends, family, and community. Few people go to their graves wishing they had put in more hours at work, but many, many people wish they had paid more attention to their friends and family.

David Myers, professor of psychology at Hope College in Holland, Michigan, has developed extensive lists of factors that can help us achieve happiness. We can't agree more with his analysis, and we believe that these lists, taken from his book *The Pursuit of Happiness: Who Is Happy, and Why*, provide invaluable insight into what we should strive to include in our lives, as well as what is less important than you might think.

So, in closing this chapter, we urge you to pay attention to the health of your mind as well as your body. Examine yourself, your personality, and your feelings. Identify the things that make you

---

### Factors that Do Not Matter for Achieving Happiness

Age
Gender
Wealth
Race
Place of residence
Parental status
Disability
Education level

*Source:* David G. Myers, *The Pursuit of Happiness*, p. 206 (Epilogue). Copyright © 1992 by the David G. and Carol P. Myers Charitable Foundation. Reprinted by permission of HarperCollins Publishers, William Morrow.

### Factors that Do Enable Happiness

Fit and healthy bodies
Realistic goals and expectations
Positive self-esteem
Feelings of control
Optimism
Outgoingness
Supportive friendships that enable companionship and confiding
A socially intimate, sexually warm, equitable marriage
Challenging work and active leisure, punctuated by adequate rest
    and retreat
A faith that entails communal support, purpose, acceptance, outward
    focus, and hope

*Source:* David G. Myers, *The Pursuit of Happiness,* p. 206 (Epilogue). Copyright ©
1992 by the David G. and Carol P. Myers Charitable Foundation. Reprinted by
permission of HarperCollins Publishers, William Morrow.

unhappy or stressed, and try to eliminate them from your life as
much as possible. Of course, you can never eliminate all the unpleas-
ant and stressful elements of your life. To reduce the negative impact
of those, find activities, such as yoga, meditation, or exercise, that relieve stress. If that doesn't work, and you find yourself depressed or
anxious, consider seeking professional help. Conversely, identify the
elements of your life that make you happy and seek to increase them.
If you can do that, you will live both a happier *and* a longer life.

## CHAPTER 7

# Tobacco: Quit Now, Here's How

When we reviewed risk factors in Chapter 3, smoking was included as one of the most common controllable risk factors for many of the top ten causes of death. We want to repeat that smoking is the single most preventable cause of death in the United States. Smoking is responsible for more than half a million deaths annually; one of every five deaths in the United States is attributed to smoking.

You might assume these are cancer deaths. While smoking is linked to at least ten different types of cancer and accounts for up to 30 percent of all cancer deaths and 85 percent of lung cancer deaths, the truth is that more smokers will die of heart disease than of cancer. Smoking is a contributing factor in up to 40 percent of all deaths due to cardiovascular disease. Smoking promotes atherosclerosis (fatty buildup in arteries), thrombosis (blood clots), coronary artery spasm, and cardiac arrhythmia. Smoking also lowers HDL cholesterol, the good cholesterol.

Furthermore, smoking is the major cause of chronic obstructive pulmonary disease (COPD), the fourth leading cause of death in the United States. COPD includes emphysema and chronic bronchitis. Perhaps you have seen people with their oxygen canisters or with a tracheotomy (hole in their neck) to aid their breathing? COPD usually afflicts patients for many years before finally suffocating them to death.

While it is true that we will all die someday, the road to death due to smoking is often a long and painful one. We know for certain that smoking damages nearly every organ in the human body.

So why would anyone smoke?

## IN DENIAL

There was a time in the 1940s and 1950s when we did not fully understand how harmful cigarettes were. It wasn't until 1964 that the effects of smoking became clear, when the Surgeon General's Advisory Committee on Smoking and Health released a 387-page report concluding that smoking causes lung cancer.

Unfortunately, and maybe due to successful advertising, 21 percent of the population still smokes in the United States. Smoking is on the rise in younger females and continues to be common among blue-collar workers.

The tobacco companies are keenly aware of how hard it is to quit smoking, so they want people to become addicted when they are young. Although advertising has become more strictly controlled in recent years, movies, television shows, and magazines still promote the "cool" image of smoking. We need to be aware of the impact of these images. The majority of adult smokers started smoking before the age of eighteen. Every day, an estimated 3,900 young people

## Media and Tobacco

Advertising has played into our cigarette habits for decades. Below are several ad campaigns from the 1940s and 1950s, when lots of people smoked. You'll notice that some of the ads allude to potential health problems by claiming their brand is a healthier choice:

"Embassy Cigarettes—Inhale to Your Heart's Content"

"Chesterfield Cigarettes—Play Safe"

"Philip Morris—An Ounce of Prevention"

"L & M Filter Tip—Just What the Doctor Ordered" (We've never ordered that in our prescription pads!)

"More Doctors Smoke Camels than Any Other Cigarette"

Remember Wayne McLaren, also known as The Marlboro Man? He was the epitome of cool . . . the rugged, handsome, independent cowboy always had a cigarette jauntily hanging from the corner of his mouth. What you might not know is that Wayne McLaren fell victim to the harmful effects of cigarette smoking and died of lung cancer in 1992. Three months before his death, he appeared at Philip Morris's annual shareholders meeting and asked the company to voluntarily limit its advertising.

Another major cigarette advertiser brought us Joe Camel, a cartoon character who was friendly, super-cool, and always having fun in his ads. The *Journal of the American Medical Association* published two reports on Joe Camel and kids. One study found that 91 percent of six-year-olds recognized Joe Camel, which is similar to the number of kids who could recognize Mickey Mouse! The other study found that Camel's share of the under-eighteen (illegal) market had risen from 0.5% to 32.8% since the start of the Joe Camel campaign less than five years before.

under the age of eighteen try their first cigarette. It's never too early to talk to the kids in your life about the devastating, lethal effects of smoking.

Amazingly, when researchers asked 1,046 smokers about the health effects of smoking, 40 percent of them didn't think their risk of lung cancer was higher than anyone else's. Clearly we still have a lot of educating to do. Remember, smoking accounts for one out of five deaths in the United States.

It is worth noting the drastic difference in cigarette use between physicians and the general public. Although 21 percent of the population smokes cigarettes, only 2 percent of physicians smoke. Maybe physicians don't smoke because they are more aware of what they are doing to their bodies, and they have seen firsthand the horrible health effects of smoking.

## WOMEN AND TOBACCO

In 1985, the American Cancer Society announced that among women, deaths due to lung cancer had surpassed deaths due to breast cancer. Since then, the lung cancer death rate has continued to climb in women. Take a look at the graph that represents deaths in women due to cancer during the last sixty years. One line represents lung cancer. The other line represents breast cancer. Notice that the breast cancer curve has stayed fairly flat, at around 25 per 100,000 women per year. Lung cancer is a different story. That line rises from almost no lung cancer in the 1930s to today's rate of about 35 deaths per 100,000 women per year.

If you smoke, now is the time to quit. Encourage smokers you know to quit. Quitting is the single best thing you can do for your health and longevity.

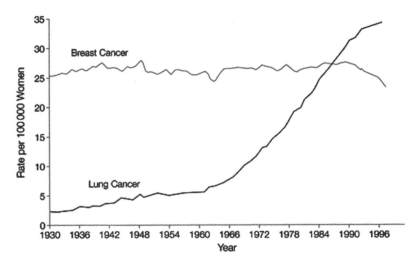

*While breast cancer gets more attention, lung cancer kills more women.*
(*Source: Women and Smoking: A Report of the Surgeon General,* 2001.)

## SECONDHAND SMOKE

People who are regularly exposed to secondhand, or "passive," smoke may be as much at risk as those who smoke cigarettes. Passive smoking increases the risk of lung cancer in nonsmokers and has also been shown to increase the risk of coronary artery disease and stroke. Researchers at Vanderbilt University reported in February 2005 that nonsmoking wives of current smokers have a 47 percent higher risk of stroke compared to wives of nonsmokers. An article published in the *British Medical Journal* in April 2005 showed that nonsmokers regularly exposed to secondhand smoke have a 25 to 73 percent greater risk of developing lung cancer, a 20 to 60 percent greater risk of developing heart disease, and a 45 to 137 percent greater risk of having a stroke than people not regularly exposed to secondhand smoke. People who worked in bars where smoking was allowed faced the greatest risk of developing disease due to second-hand smoke.

Another interesting study looked at the results of a six-month smoking ban in Helena, Montana. The number of heart attacks dropped by 40 percent after the ban was enacted. The evidence is compelling, and many cities and states across the United States have enacted smoke-free laws that ban smoking in all workplaces, restaurants, and bars. You can protect your health by choosing not to be around smokers or smoke-filled establishments.

## PIPES, CIGARS, AND SMOKELESS TOBACCO

Though cigarettes are by far the most damaging tobacco product, smoking cigars or pipes and using smokeless tobacco also increase your risk for heart disease and cancer.

Until recently, there was not much information about smokeless tobacco, which refers to chewing tobacco and snuff. However, a study published in September 2004 in the *Archives of Internal Medicine* looked at the cardiovascular risk among smokeless tobacco users. Smokeless tobacco users experience similar cardiovascular effects as cigarette smokers. These effects include an increase in heart rate (an average increase of 19 beats per minute) and blood pressure levels (up to 21 mm Hg higher systolic, and 14 mm Hg higher diastolic). Smokeless tobacco users also have higher cholesterol levels, lower HDL levels, and higher triglyceride levels than nonusers. Smokeless tobacco users also develop diabetes more often than nonusers.

The consequences of using smokeless tobacco can include cancer of the gum, mouth, pharynx, larynx, and esophagus. Worth noting, too, is that adolescents who use smokeless tobacco products are more likely to become smokers.

## Angie—Just a Few

Angie is a fifty-year-old self-described "health nut" who came in for a prevention consultation. She eats only organic foods. She exercises regularly: she does yoga and Pilates every day, as well as lifts weights and walks thirty minutes at a good pace several days each week. She gets regular physical examinations by her primary care physician, including pap smears and mammograms. She wears sunscreen and watches her cholesterol.

When asked about her family history, however, she mentioned that her parents both died of lung cancer. Angie believes that this was due to the fact that they both smoked one to two packs of cigarettes a day for nearly their entire adult lives.

When I questioned Angie about her own personal habits, I was taken aback to discover that she currently smokes! Angie smokes a pack of cigarettes a week and has been doing so for thirty years. But when she mentioned her habit, she said, "The cigarettes don't affect me. I smoke only a few cigarettes a day, and I'm extremely healthy. My doctors have always told me that all of my tests are normal. I'm not planning on quitting."

As you might imagine, I was even more surprised to hear her say that cigarettes didn't affect her, and that she didn't want to quit. I performed a physical examination, which was normal, but found that her blood pressure was slightly elevated. She went in for a heart scan (see pages 134–135) and had a score of 100, which meant that she had an elevated risk of cardiovascular disease.

Now it was Angie's turn to be shocked. "I have had lots of tests related to my health over the years and have never had any abnormal results," she told me. I was now able to show her early effects of smoking on her arteries before she had experienced any symptoms. She finally realized that smoking cigarettes was starting to affect her health. "I'll quit today," she proclaimed.

Some people believe that "just a few" cigarettes couldn't possibly do any harm or that "lung cancer won't happen to me." Quite simply, these beliefs are not true. We don't know how many cigarettes it takes to cause disease or who will die of an illness related to smoking, so the best thing to do is not smoke. Period. *−Kate Flanigan Sawyer, MD, MPH*

## What Happens to Your Body after You Quit

**20 Minutes after Quitting** Your heart rate drops.

**12 Hours after Quitting** Carbon monoxide level in your blood drops to normal.

**2 Weeks to 3 Months after Quitting** Your blood becomes less likely to clot. Your heart attack risk begins to drop. Your lung function begins to improve.

**1 to 9 Months after Quitting** Your coughing and shortness of breath decrease.

**1 Year after Quitting** Your added risk of coronary artery disease is half that of a smoker's.

**5 to 15 Years after Quitting** Your stroke risk is reduced to that of a nonsmoker.

**10 Years after Quitting** Your lung cancer death rate is about half that of a smoker's. Your risk of cancers of the mouth, throat, esophagus, bladder, kidney, and pancreas decreases.

**15 Years after Quitting** Your risk of coronary artery disease is back to that of a nonsmoker.

*Source:* U.S. Centers for Disease Control and Prevention.

We strongly recommend avoiding all forms of tobacco. Tobacco is just plain bad for your health. There is no safe level of tobacco use; even small quantities expose you to the risk of disease. Stay away from it to increase your longevity, as well as the quality of your precious years.

## QUITTING IS HARD TO DO

I (Kate Flanigan Sawyer) worked in a smoking cessation clinic at a VA Hospital during my residency. I had a patient say to me, "I've been through two wars, lost a leg, and struggled with drugs—giving up cigarettes is by far the hardest thing I have done." And I believe it. Studies have shown that the addictive effects of tobacco are similar to those of heroin and cocaine. Usually people make two or three tries, or more, before finally being able to quit. Don't give up. Even when you try to quit and fail, you will learn what helps and what doesn't. You can then use that knowledge to make a better try next time.

Some folks have success going "cold turkey." Others cut down slowly and might require the nicotine patch or gum. Many states provide hotlines or "quitlines" staffed by experienced counselors who can offer coaching and even nicotine replacements to help you quit. Several Web sites also offer great advice and support for quitting. (See page 108 for a list of Web sites.)

Whatever method you choose, we recommend that you pick a quit date sometime in the near future and stick to it!

Studies have shown that the more support you have, the better your chances for quitting. So tell your family you are quitting. Tell your friends. Tell your coworkers. Create a support network to help you stick with it.

## ADDICTED TO TASTE

Here is one method that we think can help you quit. It's a method that I (Richard J. Flanigan) published in *The American Journal of Cardiology* in 1999. It is based on the premise that people become addicted not only to nicotine, but also to taste. Most people smoke only one brand and have done so for decades.

When you are preparing to quit, the first step is to give up your favorite brand and never, ever smoke that brand again. The next step is to switch brands with every single pack you buy. This accomplishes two things: (1) it makes you buy cigarettes one pack at a time, instead

## Resources for Smoking Cessation

www.surgeongeneral.gov/tobacco
www.smoking-cessation.org/
www.nlm.nih.gov/medlineplus/smokingcessation.html
www.quitnet.com
www.americanheart.org
www.lungusa.org
National Cancer Institute Quitline (toll free) 1-877-44U-QUIT

of buying a whole carton, and (2) by changing brands often, you do not become dependent on a taste.

Do this for a month or two. Then buy your last ten packs of cigarettes, all different brands, and with decreasing amounts of tar and nicotine. Realize that the last cigarette of the last pack will be the last one you ever smoke. You can smoke these last ten packs in five days, ten days, several months, or you can drag (no pun intended) it out as long as you like. The sting to your wallet from buying ten packs at once should help remind you of the outrageous cost of this habit!

Again, whatever method works for you, we urge you to set a goal and stick to it. Believe us, quitting smoking is the single best thing you can do to improve your health.

## CHAPTER 8

# Alcohol: Friend and Foe

You may have heard that alcohol is good for you. Well, for most people, it is true. There are, indeed, significant health benefits from moderate alcohol consumption. (Moderate drinking is defined as one to two drinks per day for adult men and one drink per day for adult women.) We aren't going to encourage a nondrinker to begin drinking. However, if you do consume one or two alcoholic beverages each day, studies show that you are lowering your risk of heart disease and certain cancers.

## THE FRENCH PARADOX

Serge Renaud, MD, director of the French National Institute for Health and Medical Research, was made famous in 1991 when CBS's *60 Minutes* explored the concept of "the French paradox."

The French paradox refers to the low mortality rate from heart disease experienced by French men, despite numerous risk factors. These risk factors include high cholesterol, diabetes, hypertension, and a diet high in saturated fat. Among French men with these cardiovascular risk factors, the rate of heart disease was 40 percent less than among men in other countries with the same risk factors. This lower rate of heart disease has been attributed to a higher intake of wine, especially red wine. Many sociologists pointed out that wine drinkers tend to be less fat, they exercise more, and they drink wine only with meals, which would account for their lower risk. But when the data were examined closely, wine consumption itself was found to be a protective factor.

In fact, many of the health benefits are derived not only from red wine, but also from beer, white wine, and spirits. Over the past few years, many research studies have pointed out that the alcohol, rather than the specific components of wine, provides the protection.

In a very large study of almost twelve thousand health professionals with high blood pressure, those who consumed one alcoholic drink per day had a 32 percent lower risk of heart attack compared to those who did not drink alcohol. Studies have shown a 12 percent to 30 percent increase in HDL, the good cholesterol, with moderate consumption of alcohol. Additional studies have shown the benefits also include preventing clots, improving inflammatory status, and increasing insulin sensitivity—not to mention the stress reduction associated with moderate alcohol consumption.

Red wine does, however, impart several unique health benefits. In 2001, the American Heart Association published a Science Advisory for Healthcare Professionals entitled "Wine and Your Heart." It pointed out that red wine contains a number of plant compounds that have beneficial antioxidant properties. Among them are flavonoids, which are also present in other alcoholic beverages, such as dark beer.

Another study published in *Nature* in 2001 found that all red wines offered a benefit, but cabernet sauvignon had a slight edge over the other types of red wine. The article also pointed out that the plant compounds known as polyphenols slowed the production of a key molecule contributing to heart disease—endothelin-1.

Resveratrol is probably the most promising of the plant compounds found in red wine. It is a powerful antioxidant and has been linked to reduced heart disease in many studies. In November 2006, researchers showed that resveratrol extended the lifespan of mice by improving the function of dozens of metabolic pathways in the body.

There is some impressive evidence that grape juice also delivers health benefits since polyphenols and flavonoids are found in the skin of the red grape.

## WINE PREVENTS CANCER?

In November 2004, a group from Spain published an article in the journal *Thorax* that generated headlines around the globe because it suggested that red wine may offer some added protection against lung cancer. According to the authors, people who drank red wine had a 57 percent lower risk of developing lung cancer than people who did not drink red wine at all.

Researchers at the Fred Hutchinson Cancer Research Center in Seattle, Washington, published findings in September 2004 suggesting that a glass of red wine every day may cut a man's risk of prostate cancer in half. They found that men who consumed four or more glasses of red wine per week reduced their risk of prostate cancer by 50 percent. When they looked at aggressive prostate cancer types, there was a 60 percent lower incidence of disease. The more clinically aggressive the prostate cancer, the stronger the reduction in risk. The researchers were unable to find any significant effects— positive or negative—associated with the consumption of beer or hard liquor, and no consistent risk reduction with white wine.

So what to drink is your choice. There are benefits from all types of alcohol, but there are slightly greater benefits from drinking red wine.

## TOO MUCH OF A GOOD THING

We can't lose sight of the fact that alcohol has a dark side as well as a healthy one. The key to deriving the health benefits of alcohol lies in daily moderate consumption. For example, to consume "a week's worth" of alcohol over the course of several hours is certainly unhealthy and possibly dangerous.

Excessive alcohol consumption can lead to serious health problems. In the short term, binge drinking is a major cause of automobile accidents and acts of violence, including assault, domestic abuse, and the mistreatment of children. Long-term, excessive alcohol consumption, or alcoholism, is a major cause of death and disability, including cirrhosis of the liver, neurological problems, and stroke. It also increases the risk of certain cancers, including throat, liver, esophagus, and breast cancer. Pregnant women should never drink because of the harm it can do to the fetus. Combining prescription drugs or aspirin with alcohol can also cause significant problems and should not be done without consulting your doctor or pharmacist.

If you are like many people, however, and enjoy a glass of beer or wine in the evening, take a little extra pleasure in knowing that you are not only relaxing at the end of the day, but also improving your health and increasing your longevity. Cheers!

## CHAPTER 9

# Medications and Supplements: What to Take

In Chapters 4–8 we have discussed the many important lifestyle changes you can make to improve your health and increase your longevity. With a daily exercise routine and modifications to your diet, and by quitting smoking, you can boost your health in measurable ways. Sometimes, however, these steps are not enough to reduce your risk factors. You might need to take supplements to fill nutritional gaps or medications to bring down your blood pressure and cholesterol numbers.

Most of our patients have no problem taking medications to help relieve obvious or bothersome symptoms. Allergy pills, depression pills, pain pills, and antibiotics are among the most commonly used medicines. And most people don't mind taking those medications, because they make them feel better.

But very few of us experience the symptoms of high blood pressure and high cholesterol, so it can be difficult to understand the need to take medications to control these problems. Often we hear,

"I don't want to take medication, so what else can I do?" We understand the desire to avoid medication. No one wants to go to the pharmacy, pay the co-pay, and bring home pills that you have to remember to take on a daily basis, sometimes for years, if not for life. And then there are the side effects to deal with. But the proper medications can offer great health benefits.

On the other hand, we have patients who are not interested or don't have the willpower to make necessary lifestyle changes. They just want us to prescribe drugs to do all of the work. That's not realistic either.

The best approach for most people is to modify their diet and lifestyle and use medications if their physician determines they need additional help controlling their cholesterol and blood pressure.

We have wonderful tools to help lower the risk of heart disease and stroke. In fact, there are almost 100 different blood pressure medications and more than a dozen cholesterol-lowering medications. We will review the most commonly prescribed here so that if your physician decides you would benefit from them, you can feel confident and comfortable following that advice.

## STATINS MAY SAVE YOUR LIFE

Statins are truly remarkable medications. Many physicians consider them "miracle" drugs. They have revolutionized cardiovascular care. Introduced in 1987, statins slow the body's ability to manufacture LDL, the bad cholesterol, and increase its clearance from the bloodstream. Statins lower LDL concentrations by 18 percent to 60 percent, and reduce heart attacks by 30 percent to 60 percent and strokes by up to 50 percent. Large doses of potent statins can reduce the risk of heart attack and stroke by even more. In one study, patients who took the statin simvastatin (Zocor) and the vitamin niacin (Niaspan) reduced heart attacks, coronary death, strokes, or bypass surgery by 89 percent.

Statins dramatically reduce the risk of stroke. The MIRACL trial, published in the *Journal of the American Medical Association* in 2001, showed a 50 percent reduction in strokes among patients taking statins. A difference was seen rapidly, even in the first few days. In the recently published CARDS trial, diabetic patients who were free of heart disease but were put on a 10 mg dose of the statin drug atorvastatin calcium (Lipitor) also showed a 50 percent reduction in the number of strokes.

### Stabilizing vulnerable plaque

Statins also stabilize "vulnerable" plaque. A plaque becomes vulnerable when foam cells secrete enzymes that degrade its fibrous cap. The cap becomes thin and ruptures or is sheared off. Like tearing the scab off a cut, this exposes the interior of the plaque. Platelets collect and form a clot to begin the healing process. The size of the clot determines the outcome. If the clot is large it can occlude the vessel and cause a life-threatening heart attack or stroke. If the clot is small the healing process increases the size of the plaque.

Statins work to stabilize a plaque in five sophisticated ways. They strengthen the fibrous cap on the plaque; decrease inflammation; decrease lipid-laden foam cells; improve the function of the endothelium, the inner wall of the vessel, whose initial damage leads to plaque formation; and decrease the amount of clotting.

### Additional health benefits

Recent data have shown that statin drugs not only help lower cholesterol and improve cardiac and vascular health, but also offer some other unexpected benefits. Although the research is not as strong as that supporting statins' role in lowering cholesterol, evidence is accumulating that statins can improve other disorders, such as osteoporosis, Alzheimer's disease, multiple sclerosis, cancer, macular degeneration, and diabetes. We are waiting for more of this exciting information to be fully researched before we recommend statin use for these ailments, but we are hopeful that the preliminary reports of alternative uses for statins turn out to be valid.

### Who should take a statin and when should you start?

Again, diet and exercise are the first methods you should use to lower cholesterol and improve cardiovascular function. But if those don't succeed in getting your LDL cholesterol under 100 mg/dL, you should consider taking a statin drug. Anyone who has had a heart attack, stroke, or coronary procedure such as angioplasty or bypass should be taking a statin drug, aiming for an LDL level below 70 mg/dL.

In the June 2003 issue of the *British Medical Journal,* Drs. Nicholas Wald and Malcolm Law suggested that, due to the incredible effects of this medication, every individual should start on a low-dosage statin at age fifty-five. Dr. Robert Vogel, former chief of cardiology at the University of Maryland, agrees. In February 2005, at the Hawaii Cardiovascular Conference, he gave a talk entitled "It's Not Whether to Start a Statin, but When to Start a Statin."

When Dr. Vogel asked cardiologists at the conference who among them was taking a statin drug, almost everybody raised their hands. We have had the same experience at other conferences. Most cardiologists we know take statins. C. Richard Conti, editor of *Clinical Cardiology,* wrote in the journal's February 2007 issue that when cardiologists were surveyed at a recent meeting, 67 percent of them with one cardiovascular disease risk factor were taking statins and 33 percent with no risk factors were taking statins strictly as prevention. "Should this be a message for the general population?" he asks.

There are several statin drugs on the market. Most cardiologists feel that it does not really matter what brand you take, as long as you get your cholesterol to healthy levels. (See page 39 for our cholesterol recommendations.)

### What about side effects?

Overall, statins are extraordinarily safe—safer than aspirin and safer than many over-the-counter medications. If you are in doubt, we hope this brief discussion of the risk factors will help put you at ease.

In 1997, the U.S. Food and Drug Administration (FDA) relaxed its rules for advertising medications to consumers. Most significantly, it began allowing television advertisements. While this advertising has led to a greater awareness about medications, the FDA-mandated profiles of potential side effects have also led to fear, confusion, and concern among our patients.

Statin drugs can have some side effects, even potentially fatal ones. But, for the vast majority of people, the most common side effects they might encounter are muscle aches, nausea, diarrhea, and constipation.

Muscle discomfort is seen in up to 3 percent of patients taking a statin drug. We know of one lipid clinic that tells patients who are starting a statin drug that they will experience muscle aches, which generally go away after thirty days. In just about every case, this is exactly what happens.

A rare, but fatal, side effect due to muscle breakdown has occurred in 1.5 out of 10 million prescriptions written. To put that in perspective, there are eight million individuals in the city of New York. If they were all on a statin drug, you would expect fewer than two to die

## Muscle Aches? Take Coenzyme Q10

If you are experiencing muscle aches when taking a statin drug, our recommendation is to take 100–200 mg daily of coenzyme Q10, a supplement that's available in the vitamin aisle at drugstores and supermarkets.

Biochemically speaking, the cascade of chemical reactions that form cholesterol involves multiple steps. Statins interrupt this pathway at an early stage. Further down the line, at step nine, the pathway divides into a cholesterol-producing pathway and a coenzyme Q10–producing pathway. But because the pathway was interrupted earlier in the process, a large percentage of the coenzyme Q10 isn't made. For the majority of patients, this does not present a problem because they manage to make as much coenzyme Q10 as they need. But, some patients experience aches and pains, possibly as a result of a coenzyme Q10 deficiency.

If a patient comes to us with muscle aches and pains from taking statins, we often prescribe higher doses of coenzyme Q10. Or, we stop the statin drug, load the patient up with coenzyme Q10 for several weeks, and then restart the drug, very often with success. Talk to your doctor about what's right for you.

from this side effect. On the other hand, 2.7 million New York City residents are expected to die of heart disease or stroke, and statins could save thousands, if not a million, of them.

The other major concern with statin drugs is liver disease. Physicians should monitor liver enzymes when a patient starts a statin drug. Guidelines tell us to stop a statin drug if test results are three times their normal values. After several weeks, we can try again with the same drug at a lower dose or with a different statin.

We have seen thousands of patients on statins and only three have needed to stop the drug. Their liver function subsequently returned to normal. Fortunately, in the nearly two decades since statins were approved in the United States, there has not been a single fatality from statin-related liver disease.

We believe that, for most people, the lower cholesterol levels, the improved plaque stability, and other potential benefits greatly outweigh the risks of using statins.

## BLOOD PRESSURE MEDICATIONS

Hypertension is a major risk factor for heart disease and stroke. Clinical trials have demonstrated that by getting blood pressure to normal levels, we can reduce the incidence of stroke by up to 88 percent and of heart attack by up to 93 percent.

If you receive a high blood pressure reading, we recommend you monitor your blood pressure several times a week over a series of weeks—in your doctor's office, at home, or at the local supermarket or pharmacy. If you find that your blood pressure is consistently higher than 120/80, something needs to be done to get it under control.

Adopting a healthy lifestyle is critical to lowering your blood pressure. You can lower it with weight loss, a low-sodium diet, regular physical activity, and moderation of alcohol consumption. In fact, you can drop up to 20 mm Hg from your systolic blood pressure with about twenty pounds of weight loss. If your blood pressure is still consistently over 120/80 after about three months of lifestyle changes, it is likely that medication, in conjunction with lifestyle modifications, will be necessary to keep your blood pressure in the normal range.

Fortunately, there are many different types of medications that can help get your blood pressure under control. The five major classes of blood pressure medications available are:

1. Thiazide-type diuretics
2. Angiotensin converting enzyme inhibitors (ACE inhibitors)
3. Angiotensin receptor blockers (ARBs)
4. Calcium channel blockers
5. Beta-blockers

Thiazide-type diuretics are often the first blood pressure medications used to treat hypertension. They can be used alone or in conjunction with another class of blood pressure–lowering medications, if needed. They are inexpensive, well-studied, safe, and don't have a large list of side effects, although your physician will monitor your potassium and creatinine levels from time to time.

Angiotensin converting enzyme inhibitors (ACE inhibitors) have proven to be great blood pressure–lowering medications as well. They not only lower blood pressure, but also improve artery function and heart function, as well as protect the kidneys of people with diabetes. A common side effect of these medications is coughing (documented in 5 percent to 10 percent of people, although, in practice, we may actually see this side effect in up to 20 percent of people taking ACE inhibitors).

Angiotensin receptor blockers (ARBs) are effective blood pressure–lowering medications that are often taken by individuals who could not tolerate ACE inhibitors due to coughing.

Calcium channel blockers are also effective antihypertensive medications that help to relax the blood vessels. In the United Kingdom, these types of medications are often the first ones used to treat hypertension.

Beta-blockers were some of the earliest of the blood pressure–lowering medications. This class of drugs is effective in lowering blood pressure, but recently has fallen out of favor somewhat because of its lesser ability to protect against stroke.

## The "Polypill"—Reduce Cardiovascular Disease by 80 Percent

In June 2003, the *British Medical Journal* published an astounding article by Drs. Nicholas Wald and Malcolm Law entitled "A Strategy to Reduce Cardiovascular Disease by More than 80 Percent." They introduced the concept of the "Polypill," which is now in clinical trials, and may become mainstream soon. Drs. Wald and Law pointed out that heart disease is the largest killer in developed countries. However, if we all took the Polypill, the authors believe we could reduce heart disease by 88 percent and stroke by 80 percent—and gain eleven to twenty-four years of life span. They believe that everyone over the age of fifty-five should take it.

The Polypill is not imaginary, like the "Wonka-Vite" pill. That pill, from Roald Dahl's book *Charlie and the Great Glass Elevator,* takes twenty years off your age! The Polypill concoction includes six medications, all in low dosages and all proven to decrease heart disease and stroke. There are three medications for blood pressure (an ACE inhibitor, beta-blocker, and a diuretic), one for cholesterol (a statin), aspirin, and folic acid.

There is excellent evidence to indicate that the Polypill could work to dramatically decrease the incidence of heart disease and stroke. Until it hits the shelves, however, we often recommend to our patients a medication regimen quite similar to the Polypill.

### The "Polymeal": Maybe a better idea?

Several months after the original Polypill article was published, another article in the *British Medical Journal* addressed the same concept. This one was entitled "The Polymeal: A More Natural, Safer, and Probably Tastier (than the Polypill) Strategy." This article outlined an alternative strategy that researchers believe could reduce cardiovascular disease by more than 75 percent. The authors point out how the Polypill is promising in terms of cardiovascular risk management, but they have reviewed the literature and feel that this risk reduction could also be achieved by eating foods that are proven to prevent heart disease, stroke, and cancer. The Polymeal consists of wine, fish, dark chocolate, fruits and vegetables, garlic, and almonds. Sounds pretty good, doesn't it?

We bet that a combination of the Polymeal and the Polypill could essentially eradicate heart disease on this planet!

Your physician will decide which class or combination of blood pressure–lowering medications is best for you, based on your health status and risk factors.

## ASPIRIN—OVER A CENTURY AS A MIRACLE DRUG

Who would have known that a tiny pill costing just a few pennies could have such a large impact on your longevity? Aspirin has been touted as the wonder drug by many physicians.

Aspirin is certainly not a new drug. In fact, the active compound found in aspirin has been used since the time of Hippocrates, more than two thousand years ago. At that time, it was given in the form of a powder made from the bark and leaves of the willow tree. In the early 1800s, the active ingredient in willow bark was extracted and developed into a pure state—salicylic acid. In 1899, Felix Hoffmann, a German chemist who worked for Bayer, was looking for a remedy for his father, who was suffering from arthritis. He treated the salicylic acid with a buffer to protect the stomach and came up with aspirin (acetylsalicylic acid). Bayer patented and marketed the drug, and, within a year, aspirin was the number-one drug in the world.

Aspirin has been around for so long that researchers have been able to study this drug in depth. Our knowledge about aspirin as a potential cardiac lifesaver began more than fifty years ago. In 1948, Dr. Lawrence Craven, a general practitioner in California, noted that the four hundred men he prescribed aspirin to had not suffered heart attacks. He started to recommend aspirin regularly to his patients and colleagues. An aspirin a day, he believed, could dramatically reduce the risk of heart attack. Many studies done since then have confirmed Dr. Craven's findings.

In 1988, the FDA approved aspirin to reduce the risk of recurrent heart attack and to prevent the first heart attack in patients with unstable angina (atypical chest pain). Aspirin was also approved to prevent recurrent transient ischemic attacks (TIAs, or "mini-strokes") in men. All men who had suffered previous strokes were also approved for daily aspirin therapy. Over the next decade, researchers continued to find more use and value in aspirin for both men and women. In 1998, the FDA updated and expanded its recommendations for aspirin therapy.

Aspirin is currently approved by the FDA for:

1. Reducing the risk of complications or death during a suspected heart attack
2. Preventing a recurrent transient ischemic stroke, or TIA, in men and women
3. Reducing the risk of recurrent heart attack and stroke
4. Reducing the risk of recurrent blockage for those who have had heart bypass surgery or other procedures to clear blocked arteries

No wonder it's not just used as a pain reliever! In fact, according to aspirin manufacturer Bayer, more people take aspirin to reduce their risk of heart disease than to treat minor aches and pains.

### How does aspirin work to reduce heart disease?

Some blockages in our arteries are caused by blood clots that travel through the bloodstream and get wedged in a coronary artery, and some blockages are due to the buildup of plaque in our arteries. Aspirin works in both types of blockages by reducing the clotting ability of platelets. It decreases the chance of clot formation and reduces the ability of platelets to block arteries narrowed by built-up plaque.

A newer theory about the cause of cardiovascular disease posits that inflammation in the artery can also lead to narrowing and hardening of the arteries. Aspirin may help lower the risk of heart disease by reducing inflammation in the blood vessels themselves.

### Should I take it?

Although aspirin is known to have many positive benefits and is regarded as a safe and inexpensive preventive measure, aspirin therapy is not for everyone. Aspirin has side effects, like any medication. As explained above, aspirin helps decrease clotting. In some people, a diminished clotting ability can lead to a risk of excessive bleeding. This can happen anywhere in your body, including the brain, which causes stroke, and the stomach, which causes ulcers. The risk of bleeding increases with increasing doses of aspirin and when it is used in combination with nonsteroidal anti-inflammatory drugs (ibuprofen, Advil, Naproxen, to name a few) or oral anticoagulants (such as Coumadin). There are also small but significant risks of liver damage, hearing loss or ringing in the ears, allergic reaction, and breathing problems. We recommend you discuss taking aspirin with your physician, who can help you decide if the benefits would outweigh the risks.

Most people will not have significant problems with aspirin therapy under the supervision of a physician. In fact, one doctor who headed one of the largest studies on aspirin believes that it should be used by "just about everyone" who has survived a heart attack or stroke due to a blocked blood vessel, as well as those who have had symptoms of an evolving heart attack within the previous twenty-four hours. The American Heart Association recommends that anyone who has already had a heart attack or stroke should take aspirin to prevent another event.

Remember, however, that aspirin alone is not enough to prevent cardiovascular disease. Aspirin is not a substitute for a healthy lifestyle or other risk-lowering medications. It should be used in conjunction with a well-rounded prevention program and in consultation with your doctor.

### How much should I take?

Amazingly, even though it is such a wonder drug and has been around so long, the best preventive dose of aspirin is still controversial. One of the first, largest, and most convincing trials to document aspirin's benefits was the Physicians' Health Study, released almost twenty years ago. This study showed a 44 percent decrease in heart attacks among those physicians who took 325 mg of aspirin every other day.

Next, researchers looked at varying doses of aspirin to see if lower amounts would be just as effective. One study of forty thousand women over forty-five found that a small dose of aspirin (100 mg every other day) reduced the risk of a first stroke by nearly 25 percent. The same types of results were found in studies of men taking aspirin. Since then, there have been many studies that support aspirin at doses of 75–150 mg as being at least as effective as higher daily doses.

Our advice for men and women over the age of fifty is to take two baby aspirin or half of a regular aspirin (162 mg) each day, unless there is a tendency for bleeding or bruising.

### Aspirin and cancer

There has been some recent buzz about aspirin and cancer prevention. Wouldn't it be wonderful if the pill you were taking to prevent heart attacks and strokes also helped prevent cancers? Aspirin just may do that. Preliminary studies have suggested that aspirin may reduce the risk of several major cancers, including colon, breast, prostate, lung, esophagus, stomach, bladder, and ovarian cancer. The cancer-preventive benefits of aspirin are not proven yet, and we will have to wait for more definitive studies to see if the promising initial findings are indeed true.

## SUPPLEMENTS—JUST A FEW

Not many people can afford to spend $500 a month on various supplements, enzymes, and vitamins—and we don't know anyone who should!

After a thorough search of the literature on supplements, we have been able to narrow our recommendations to just a few. We were specifically looking for well-designed studies in peer-reviewed medical journals, not self-published, company-sponsored studies. There's a lot of data out there, not all of it valid. Most supplements' claims are unregulated, and many are backed by little or no evidence.

---

### Don't Take Too Much of These

**Vitamin A acetate or palmitate (retinol).** It can increase the risk of hip fractures, liver abnormalities, and birth defects.

**Vitamin E.** Recent studies show that, in high doses, it does not protect against heart disease, stroke, or dementia, and can actually be detrimental to your health. To be safe, take no more than 200 IU per day.

**Iron.** Too much can cause constipation or iron overload.

**Zinc.** It can depress your immune system.

---

Supplements are just that—supplements. They are not intended to take the place of the foods we eat, but to be used in conjunction with a healthy diet. No supplement can substitute for good eating habits, physical activity, smoking cessation, or weight loss as a means of minimizing your risk of heart disease or cancer. We recommend getting the nutrition, antioxidants, vitamins, and minerals that you need primarily from your diet. Some supplements, however, can help fill "gaps" in your diet.

### Multivitamins

For starters, we recommend that everyone take a multivitamin daily as a type of "dietary insurance." That's all you should expect from your multivitamin. A daily multivitamin is not a magic bullet. There is no good evidence that vitamins give you energy, improve your athletic performance, reduce stress, or burn fat. But a regular multivitamin is important to help supplement your diet because even a healthy diet can sometimes lack necessary nutrients. A multivitamin is a cheap and easy way to round out a healthy diet.

Hundreds of types of multivitamins are available on the market, and it can be extremely confusing to choose the "right" one. Some multivitamins have too little of one thing and too much of another, which can lead to adverse health effects. You are generally safe if you stay at or below the daily value (DV) or recommended dietary allowance (RDA) for each ingredient in your multivitamin. Always check the label for amounts. It is especially important to get adequate amounts of B complex, folic acid, and selenium. In fact, there are many good multivitamins on the market—and you don't need to spend a fortune. Many large supermarket and drugstore chains carry their own brand of multivitamin, which are formulated to copy major national brands. Many of them are inexpensive and their ingredients meet the recommendations.

### Calcium and vitamin D

Calcium and vitamin D are important for strengthening your bones, particularly as you age. Research has shown that in individuals over sixty, calcium and vitamin D increase bone density and can lower the risk of hip fracture.

Calcium is often too bulky to fit the daily value into a multivitamin, so you will likely need to obtain your calcium from another source. We recommend you take a supplement unless you get enough from your diet. You need 1,000 mg of calcium daily from ages nineteen to fifty, and 1,200 mg of calcium daily if you are over fifty. Men should not take more than 1,500 mg a day.

You also may want to make sure you're getting enough vitamin D, as a multivitamin may not have the amount you need. Sometimes a calcium supplement will also contain vitamin D—check the label for amounts. You need 400 IU of daily vitamin D if you are between fifty and seventy years old. If you are over seventy, you need 600–1,000 IU per day.

### Vitamin E

The research on vitamin E has been inconsistent over the past several years. Many studies have disagreed on whether vitamin E protects against heart disease. In 2003, a comprehensive study looked at the largest and best-designed vitamin E trials to see if the confusion could be cleared up. In the end, it was found that vitamin E does not provide any benefit in decreasing the risk of heart disease or stroke, and researchers concluded that the routine use of vitamin E was not supported.

### Fish oil capsules

Simply put, omega-3 fatty acids are good for your heart. (See pages 79–83 for more information.) These fatty acids can be obtained through a diet rich in plant and fish oils, with fish and fish oils containing the most powerful fatty acids EPA (eicosapentaenoic acid) and DHA (docosahexaenoic acid). They not only reduce cardiovascular risk, they also decrease risk for heart rhythm disorders, which can lead to sudden death, and blood clotting, which can lead to heart attack and stroke.

The American Heart Association recommends adults eat fish (salmon, sardines, mackerel, herring, tuna, trout) at least two times a week. However, if you do not eat fish, we recommend you take fish oil capsules. Take one a day, or as many as three a day, depending on your risk of heart disease and the amount prescribed by your physician. Also, remember to read the manufacturer's label, since not all capsules contain the same amount of omega-3 fatty acids.

Remember, vitamins and supplements are not a replacement for a well-balanced diet. Know what you are taking and the risks associated with overuse, especially for those mentioned above.

## CHAPTER 10

# Simple Tests:
# Monitor Your Health

Screening for disease is crucial. Screening tests can often detect a disease, such as cancer, before you experience symptoms. Early detection will allow you to begin early treatment, which vastly improves your chances of successfully treating it. By the time you experience symptoms, the disease has already developed and could be severe or even deadly. Screening tests can also detect early changes warning of increased risk for disease. Thus alerted, you can modify your lifestyle or medication to help prevent disease before it develops. Below, we recommend several screening tests for the diseases most likely to kill you.

## HEART DISEASE AND STROKE

The ability of medical tests to detect the early onset of cardiovascular disease has improved dramatically in the past decade. Many of the tests available today can detect cardiovascular disease in its earliest stages—many years before a heart attack or stroke would occur.

There is no stand-alone test that provides *all* the information you need to understand the status of your arteries. But each test can contribute a piece of the puzzle to help create a complete picture of your arterial health. We believe that gathering as much information as you can about yourself and your health is extremely valuable. If you find several abnormalities on screening tests, you will likely be more aggressive about controlling your risk factors.

### Cholesterol (lipid) panel

This test measures levels of several different fats in your blood: total cholesterol; high-density lipoprotein (HDL); low-density lipoprotein (LDL); and triglycerides.

*Recommendations:* Get this test each decade, starting in your teens, until age fifty. After fifty, get this test at least every five years, or more often if you have any abnormalities; if there are changes in

---

### An Important Longevity Partner: Your Physician

One of the most important elements of an effective longevity plan is a good relationship with your physician. Your doctor can help you define your risk factors by taking a medical history, performing a physical examination, and running routine blood tests. He or she can note year-to-year changes in your health and risk factors, and recommend specific tests based on findings from your visit. It is well worth your time to find a physician you like and see him or her every year. Your life could depend on it.

---

your health status, such as weight gain; if you are taking lipid-lowering medications; or as recommended by your health-care provider.

National guidelines call for total cholesterol under 200 mg/dL, HDL cholesterol greater than 45 mg/dL, LDL cholesterol under 100 mg/dL, and triglycerides under 150 mg/dL. We believe these are minimum requirements, and suggest more ambitious goals to arrest and reverse disease. The optimal scores for men and women are 150 mg/dL total cholesterol, HDL greater than 50 mg/dL, LDL below 70 mg/dL, and triglycerides less than 100 mg/dL. Your cholesterol/HDL ratio should be less than 3.0. If you can achieve these numbers, you will not develop atherosclerosis.

### Advanced lipid testing: LDL and HDL particle size and Lp(a)

The advanced lipid testing takes the information provided from the standard test and breaks it down into even more valuable components, telling you more about the quality of your cholesterol.

The test looks at the size of the LDL and HDL particles. Large LDL and HDL particles are preferable to small ones. The smaller the LDL particle, the more atherogenic, or heart damaging, it is. Large LDLs are much less dangerous because they have difficulty slipping through the lining of the blood vessel to develop into a plaque. The same concept holds true for HDL; bigger HDL particles are more effective at clearing cholesterol from the bloodstream. Knowing the nature of your LDL and HDL particles gives you a good idea of how aggressive you need to be in managing your lipids.

Fortunately, weight loss, exercise, medications (if needed), and a healthy diet can improve these values significantly.

The other component of the advanced test is Lp(a)—a separate atherogenic lipoprotein, which is genetically determined. An elevated Lp(a) level is a marker associated with higher cardiovascular risk.

*Recommendations:* Get advanced lipid testing at age forty-five for males and age fifty-five for females if you have no risk factors and normal lipids. If your lipids are abnormal, you should consider getting this advanced test earlier, perhaps five years earlier. This test is now available nationwide in standard laboratories. You want to have more large, type A, LDL particles than small, type B, particles. You want more of the large HDL-2 particles than the small HDL-3 particles. You want your Lp(a) to come in at less than 30 mg/dL.

### Heart scan: Coronary artery calcium testing

A heart scan is a quick, safe, and easy test done in one breath. The scan detects and measures calcium that collects at the site of an arterial plaque in your coronary arteries. It measures the extent of your artery disease, known as plaque burden, and serves as a valuable predictor of future cardiac events. This test picks up early disease long before symptoms occur and, thus, can demonstrate the need for aggressive prevention. We believe this is one of the most valuable tests to evaluate cardiovascular risk.

This test is also highly motivating. The heart scan produces an image that actually shows the calcium buildup in the coronary arteries. Patients who see that image can better comprehend that they have disease and will often become very motivated to implement prevention strategies.

People with a score of 0 on a heart scan have no detectable calcium, thus no atherosclerosis, and an excellent long-term prognosis for heart disease. A study published in *The American Journal of Cardiology* quantified the risks associated with increasing heart calcium scores. Researchers performed heart scans on more than 2,200 people with no evidence of heart disease, then reevaluated them seven to nine years later. The presence of *any* calcium increased the patients' risk of developing heart disease. When the score rose to 50–99, the risk of heart disease doubled. People with scores of 100–199 had 3.8 times the risk of heart disease as those with a 0 score, and those with scores of 200–399 had 9.8 times the risk. Scores of greater than 2,000 were associated with a whopping 55.7-fold increase in the risk of cardiovascular disease.

***Recommendations:*** All men over forty-five and women over fifty-five should get a calcium scan or a carotid artery wall thickness measurement (CIMT, see pages 138–139).

Any score greater than 0 suggests that you have some atherosclerosis and should consider lifestyle changes to stop further development of disease. For those with a score greater than 80, we recommend an aggressive prevention program that would likely include a statin medication to reduce plaque.

### Inflammatory markers: hs-CRP and Lp-PLA2

Scientists have become aware in recent years that inflammation plays a large role in cardiovascular events. A series of blood tests now available for those at higher risk can detect proteins, called inflammatory markers, that signal the presence of inflammation. Numerous studies have connected high-sensitivity C-reactive protein (hs-CRP) with coronary artery disease and heart attacks. A newer marker, lipoprotein-associated phospholipase A2 (Lp-PLA2), is an excellent marker more specific for *vascular* inflammation as it is secreted by foam cells, the fat-laden inflammatory cells in the arterial wall. These cells render the plaque vulnerable to rupture. There is a direct relationship between the amount of Lp-PLA2 and the risk for heart attack and stroke.

The good news is that both of these inflammatory markers can be decreased with exercise, no smoking, and statin drugs.

*Recommendations:* Test for inflammatory markers once at forty-five for males, fifty-five for females, then every decade if normal; if abnormal, retest to confirm, then monitor periodically. For hs-CRP, less than 1 mg/L indicates a low risk of heart attack, and 1–3 mg/L is average risk. If you have more than 4 mg/L, you are at high risk for a heart attack. For Lp-PLA2, you want to have a reading of less than 235 mg/dL, which indicates minimal inflammation in your arteries.

### Electrocardiogram (EKG or ECG)

The electrocardiogram is a simple and inexpensive test that provides a quick picture of your heart's electrical function, which controls the beating of your heart.

An excellent article in the March 7, 2007, issue of the *Journal of the American Medical Association* points out the value of routine EKG testing. The researchers did a routine EKG on 14,749 postmenopausal women with no symptoms of heart disease. They divided the women into three groups based on their EKGs: those whose EKGs were normal, those with minor abnormalities, and those with major abnormalities. The researchers followed the women for an average of 5.2 years and noted the frequency of cardiac events. They found that those with normal EKG readings had 21 heart attacks per 10,000 women. Those with minor abnormalities had 40 events per 10,000 women. The group with major abnormalities at baseline had 75 events per 10,000 women, a greater than threefold increase in the number of heart attacks experienced by women with normal EKGs. Although this research was done only on women, it applies to men as well.

Additionally, a baseline EKG can be very valuable for future comparison when changes occur. As cardiologists, we are always amazed

## Simple Advice for You at All Ages

**Age 0 to 40**—The major thrust for these years is to prevent disease from occurring in the first place. Screening is valuable, but at this young age, we recommend that you focus on lifestyle modification practices (not smoking, watching your diet, and exercising regularly)—unless you are at higher than normal risk for certain diseases.

**Age 40 to 55**—The focus during this time is on detecting early signs of disease and arresting further development of disease. We recommend getting baseline readings on most of the screening tests we have outlined in this chapter.

**Age 55+**—This is the period of time that disease often shows up. So, the focus at this age is on detecting and reversing disease. We recommend repeating the baseline tests (done at age forty-five) to evaluate for further progression of disease. Also, focus on aggressive prevention—it is never too late to practice prevention.

at the incidence of "silent heart attacks," which represent approximately 10 percent to 15 percent of all heart attacks. Patients don't feel the classic "elephant on the chest" pain, and usually don't seek medical attention. When they come in for a routine visit, however, their EKGs have changed. (Heart attacks leave very clear changes on the EKG tracings.) On careful questioning, many of these patients mention a bout of discomfort, which they passed off as "indigestion," but which was actually a heart attack. These individuals are at much higher risk for another heart attack and need an aggressive prevention program. The baseline EKG provides a valuable reference point, which helps cardiologists detect the changes that signal a silent heart attack and the need for aggressive prevention.

*Recommendations:* Get a baseline EKG when you are forty years old if you are a man, fifty years old if you are a woman.

### Treadmill stress testing

A treadmill stress test monitors your heart while you exercise to your maximum ability. EKG leads are hooked up to your chest while you run on the treadmill in intervals of increasing speed and elevation. Changes in the EKG pattern indicate reduced blood flow due to artery blockages. A treadmill stress test not only looks at EKG changes, but also has other valuable measurements that predict risk, such as exercise capacity, arrhythmias, and heart rate recovery.

*Recommendations:* We advocate routine treadmill stress testing for men by age forty-five and for women by age fifty-five.

### Carotid ultrasound

The carotid arteries, which run up the sides of the neck and supply blood to the brain, are a very common source of clots that cause stroke. A physical examination with a stethoscope can detect some blockages in the carotid arteries. But we have been astounded by how many times a carotid ultrasound detects an extensive blockage that was not heard with a stethoscope. Ultrasound uses high-frequency sound waves to produce an image of your arteries.

Some ultrasound machines can also measure the thickness of the carotid artery walls, known as carotid intima media thickness (CIMT). Thick artery walls are usually ones filled with sclerotic plaques. The technology of this particular measurement is very sophisticated, and not all ultrasound machines have this capability. But if it is available, it is an excellent measurement of vascular age. Thicker carotid artery walls have been linked to both stroke and heart disease.

*Recommendations:* We advise all men and women over the age of sixty to get a carotid ultrasound. If it is normal, we recommend repeating it in ten years. If it is abnormal, we recommend yearly ultrasounds to monitor change and the effects of medications and lifestyle modifications.

Men over forty-five, women over fifty-five, and anyone with cardiovascular disease risk factors should get a CIMT test if it is available.

### Heart ultrasound: An echocardiogram

An echocardiogram is an ultrasound of the heart. This test evaluates the structure of the heart, its valves, and their functions. It shows whether the valves leak or not, and it also looks at the heart's pumping ability, known as ejection fraction, and at the filling pattern of the heart.

This is a particularly valuable test for people with high blood pressure. High blood pressure can cause the muscle of the heart to become enlarged, a process called hypertrophy. This can affect the pumping and filling of the heart. With proper blood pressure medication, this hypertrophy can be minimized and even reversed.

*Recommendations:* Men with hypertension should get this test at age forty-five; women with hypertension should get this test at age fifty-five.

### Abdominal aorta ultrasound

An abdominal aortic aneurysm is a weakness in the wall of your aorta, the largest blood vessel in the body, which carries blood from your heart to the lower part of your body. That weakness leads to a bulge or "out-pouching" of the vessel, called an aneurysm. An aortic aneurysm can suddenly rupture, and the result is almost always fatal.

Men are much more likely to have abdominal aortic aneurysms than women. These types of aneurysms are most likely to occur in people who smoke or have smoked.

The key is to detect the presence of this aneurysm before it ruptures. Sometimes, you or your physician can feel the aneurysm on a physical examination. But aortic aneurysms often go undetected. An abdominal ultrasound test measures the size of your aorta and is the best test to show whether it is dangerous and in need of repair.

*Recommendations:* Every male over sixty who currently smokes or has a history of smoking should be screened. Everyone should be screened after the age of sixty-five.

### Ankle-brachial index (ABI) test

This is a simple, quick test done to screen for peripheral arterial disease of the legs. This test is done by measuring blood pressure at the ankle and in the arm while you are at rest, and sometimes after exercise.

The ankle-brachial index (the ankle blood pressure divided by the arm blood pressure) is used to predict the severity of peripheral arterial disease.

*Recommendations:* All men at age forty-five and women at age fifty-five should get a baseline ankle-brachial index screening. If it is normal, repeat in five years. If it is abnormal, consult with your physician and have it done more frequently.

A normal resting ankle-brachial index is 1 or 1.1. This means that the blood pressure in your lower extremity is the same or greater than the pressure in your arm, and there is no significant obstruction of blood flow. A resting ankle-brachial index of less than 1 is abnormal, with an index of less than 0.5 indicating a severe obstruction of blood flow.

## CANCER

Below is a figure that shows the most prevalent types of cancer in men and women. You can see that lung cancer is well ahead of all others for both men and women. The second most common types of cancer are the "gender" cancers, breast for women and prostate for men. This is followed by colon and rectum cancers in both men and women. These top four types of cancer account for almost 60 percent of all cancers. This is where we should put our preventive emphasis.

Just as a side note, it is interesting that many women surveyed about cancer were more concerned with breast cancer than any other. But lung cancer is far more prevalent in women than breast cancer. The campaign for breast cancer has been fantastic. We are all aware of the breast cancer symbols: the Race for the Cure, the pink ribbon. What type of awareness is out there for women and lung cancer? The tobacco industry must be pleased.

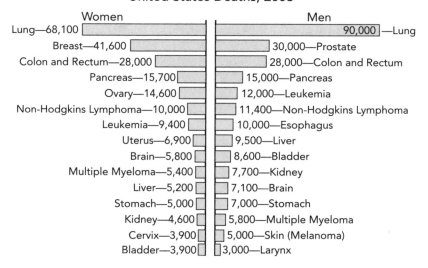

### Leading Cancer Killers
### United States Deaths, 2003

| Women | Men |
|---|---|
| Lung—68,100 | 90,000—Lung |
| Breast—41,600 | 30,000—Prostate |
| Colon and Rectum—28,000 | 28,000—Colon and Rectum |
| Pancreas—15,700 | 15,000—Pancreas |
| Ovary—14,600 | 12,000—Leukemia |
| Non-Hodgkins Lymphoma—10,000 | 11,400—Non-Hodgkins Lymphoma |
| Leukemia—9,400 | 10,000—Esophagus |
| Uterus—6,900 | 9,500—Liver |
| Brain—5,800 | 8,600—Bladder |
| Multiple Myeloma—5,400 | 7,700—Kidney |
| Liver—5,200 | 7,100—Brain |
| Stomach—5,000 | 7,000—Stomach |
| Kidney—4,600 | 5,800—Multiple Myeloma |
| Cervix—3,900 | 5,000—Skin (Melanoma) |
| Bladder—3,900 | 3,000—Larynx |

*Source:* National Center for Health Statistics.

This next chart describes the five-year survival rates of patients diagnosed with these top four cancers and treated before the cancer spread. The survival rates for these cancers have improved over the past twenty-five to thirty years. In fact, the survival rates are over 80 percent for lung, prostate, breast, and colorectal cancers that have been detected early. In contrast, on the right side of the same chart, you can see that people diagnosed with cancer that has spread from its primary site, called metastatic cancer, have very poor survival rates.

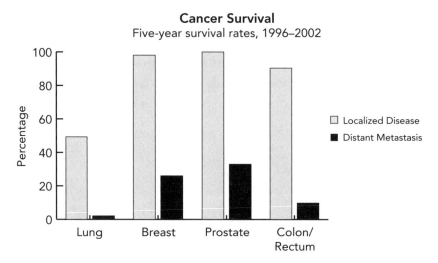

*This graph clearly demonstrates that early detection of cancer increases the number of years you can expect to survive.* (*Source:* National Cancer Institute.)

The point is, get your cancer screening tests and get them regularly so that you can detect these diseases early in their development when chances of survival are much better.

Although early detection vastly improves your odds of surviving cancer, too many people in the United States fail to screen for cancer.

The American Cancer Society reported on the prevalence of screening among people *with* health insurance. Of these, only 42 percent of individuals over the age of fifty have had a sigmoidoscopy or colonoscopy. In women forty and older, only 58 percent have had a mammogram. Only 54 percent of men have had a PSA test for prostate cancer.

There are tons of excuses for not getting screened, including many limitations in the current health-care system. But remember, the key to cancer survival is early detection. And the way to detect cancer early is through screening. We do not want you to develop a life-threatening case of cancer because you failed to get a screening test. Screening is critical. Get it done!

***Recommendations:*** In 2006, the American Cancer Society published recommendations for the early detection of cancer in average-risk, asymptomatic people. We support these guidelines and recommend that you consider their valuable information. Of course, if you are at high risk for these cancers, have a significant family history, or are experiencing symptoms, your physician may recommend additional or more frequent testing.

**Breast**—Start with a yearly clinical breast exam at age twenty. Begin yearly mammograms at age forty.

**Colorectal**—Get a colonoscopy at age fifty, then once every ten years.

**Prostate**—Test for prostate-specific antigen (PSA) and have a digital rectal examination at age fifty—earlier if you have risk factors—then annually thereafter.

**Lung**—The jury is still out on CT screening for lung cancer. While one study demonstrated improved survival among those whose cancer was detected early by CT scans, another study indicated that CT scans resulted in more cancer diagnoses and treatments, but did not necessarily reduce deaths from cancer. We recommend that smokers over forty discuss CT scanning with their physicians.

## COPD

### Spirometry

Chronic bronchitis and emphysema, the two main elements of chronic obstructive pulmonary disease, don't strike suddenly, but develop slowly over many years. By the time people feel short enough of breath to seek help, they have often lost half their lung function. Pulmonary function tests, also called spirometry, can detect abnormalities in your lung function before you notice any significant symptoms.

There is no cure for COPD, but you can extend your life by quitting smoking and getting supplemental oxygen if you need it. And you can greatly improve the quality of your life if you get proper treatment for COPD. The real goal, however, is not getting the disease. Quitting smoking is the first place to start.

*Recommendations:* If you have a history of smoking tobacco, have had significant occupational exposure to dust or pollutants, or have had significant exposure to secondhand smoke, we recommend regular pulmonary function tests to detect disease and monitor changes over time.

## ACCIDENTS

### Bone density screening

Bone density screening is an important test related to falls. People with low bone density are more likely to suffer fractures when they fall down. Osteopenia refers to mildly low bone density, while lower bone density is called osteoporosis. Bone density screening is a simple, noninvasive, and painless test. If you learn that you have either osteopenia or osteoporosis, you can make lifestyle changes and take medications to slow bone loss and possibly even increase your bone density.

**Recommendations:** Women are much more likely than men to suffer osteoporosis. All women at sixty-five and men at seventy should get a baseline bone density screening. You should get screened earlier, if you break a bone or if your physician recommends it. If you have normal bone density, then retest in five to ten years. If you have either osteopenia or osteoporosis, then retest every two years or more often, as recommended by your physician.

## TYPE 2 DIABETES

### Fasting plasma glucose

A fasting plasma glucose blood test determines how much sugar is in your blood. If your blood sugar is too high, that means that you either do not have enough insulin or that your cells are not responding to it. In either case, a high blood glucose level can indicate that you have either diabetes or pre-diabetes.

**Recommendations:** Anyone over forty-five should be tested, particularly if you are overweight (if your BMI is above 25; see chart on page 48). If you are under forty-five, but overweight, and have a risk factor for diabetes, such as lack of physical activity or family history, you should be tested now. If your blood glucose level is normal, repeat the test in one to three years.

You want your level to be under 100 mg/dL. A fasting blood glucose level between 100 and 125 mg/dL signals pre-diabetes or impaired fasting glucose and a 54 percent increased chance of having a heart attack. A person with a fasting blood glucose level of 126 mg/dL or higher has diabetes, which decreases longevity by an average of fifteen years.

## KIDNEY DISEASE

Symptoms of renal disease don't really appear until kidney disease has progressed. Screening is important to detect disease and begin early treatment, if needed.

### Blood tests

Tests of your blood urea nitrogen (BUN), creatinine, and glomerular filtration rate (GFR) measure how efficiently the kidneys are filtering waste from the blood. Abnormalities can signal poor kidney function and disease.

### Urine tests

Urine tests measure the amount of a protein called albumin in the urine. A large amount of protein, known as proteinuria, is a sign of kidney damage.

*Recommendations:* Kidney disease is caused mainly by diabetes, hypertension, and cardiovascular disease. If you have any of these conditions, or a family history of kidney disease, test annually. Otherwise, both men and women should start screening at age forty-five, or earlier if recommended by your physician.

## PNEUMONIA/INFLUENZA, ALZHEIMER'S, SEPTICEMIA

There are no routine tests available for prevention or early detection of these diseases. If you have concerns, talk to your physician.

## CHAPTER 11

# Longevity Made Simple: Putting It All Together

Here are ten tips, in order of importance, that can make a measurable difference in your health and longevity. Follow these tips, and increase your odds of living a long, disease-free life.

1. **Lower cholesterol.** Heart disease is the number one cause of death, but it doesn't occur if your total cholesterol is 150 mg/dL or less. The goal we should shoot for is 150 mg/dL total cholesterol, with 70 mg/dL LDL and 50 mg/dL HDL. That may seem extreme, given that the average cholesterol levels in the United States are 209 mg/dL for men and 225 mg/dL for women. However, they are completely achievable as evidenced by the fact that many populations around the world have average cholesterol levels of 125 mg/dL to 140 mg/dL.

If you can't achieve these numbers with diet and exercise, you should strongly consider one of the statin class of cholesterol-lowering medications. These medications are truly miracle drugs that can prevent up to 60 percent of heart events and 50 percent of strokes.

They decrease inflammation, prevent clots, and stabilize artery plaques, and they seem to be beneficial for numerous other conditions, including Alzheimer's disease and macular degeneration.

2. **Lower blood pressure.** Stroke is the number three killer in the United States and causes the most disability. If a stroke doesn't kill you, it is likely to leave you unable to speak or move well. A very large number of strokes can be prevented by maintaining a normal blood pressure of 120/80 mm Hg or lower. People with systolic blood pressure of 180 die of heart disease nine times more frequently than people with blood pressure of 120, and they die thirteen times more often of stroke. Increasing blood pressure from 120 to just 139, considered by many to be borderline high blood pressure, doubles to quadruples vascular events. Diet, exercise, and medications are your best tools to lower blood pressure.

3. **Avoid tobacco.** Eliminating tobacco from your life is the single best preventive measure you can take. Each cigarette takes an average of seven minutes off your life. And being exposed to cigarette smoke is almost as bad as smoking. There was a 40 percent decrease in heart attacks in Helena, Montana, when the city enacted a non-smoking policy.

4. **Eat a diet rich in fish, fruit, and vegetables**. Two servings of fish each week cut heart disease by 38 percent to 67 percent and reduce sudden cardiac death by 50 percent. Sudden cardiac death decreases up to 81 percent when fish or a fish oil capsule (1 gram) is consumed daily. The main component of cancer prevention is a diet rich in multicolored vegetables, which contain unique antioxidants and polyphenols. The Mediterranean diet has been shown to prolong life, decrease Alzheimer's disease, and decrease heart disease up to 76 percent.

5. **Get exercise.** It does all the right things for the body, the mind, and the biochemistry. It is the best way to keep your immune system in tune. You just have to do it. How much? Thirty minutes a day of

walking will prevent 20 percent to 50 percent of many diseases, including heart disease, sudden cardiac death, some cancers, and osteoporosis, to name a few.

6. **Maintain a healthy weight**. Two-thirds of the U.S. population are overweight. Obesity and diabetes have skyrocketed in the past ten years. Eat like the Okinawans, the longest-living people on the planet: eat slowly and stop when you are 80 percent full. Give your brain enough time to register that your stomach is full. Also, use smaller plates (for portion control), and enjoy a sensible mid-morning and mid-afternoon snack to keep from getting hungry.

7. **Prevent accidents**. Accidents are the fifth leading cause of fatalities. The highest mortality from accidents is due to motor vehicles, yet 50 percent of teenagers don't wear seat belts. So be smart and buckle up before you drive, and make sure your teens buckle up too. Prevent falls by accident-proofing your home, especially the bathroom, as most falls happen in the shower. And be extra careful when using a ladder!

8. **Drink alcohol**. We know it seems hard to believe, but just about every study undertaken confirms that a *small* amount of alcohol daily provides a substantial (30 percent to 50 percent) benefit in decreasing heart disease. We suggest a glass of red wine because of the beneficial properties of the skin of the red grape, which contains polyphenols, resveratrol, and antioxidants.

9. **Take aspirin**. Just like statins and fish oil capsules, aspirin is truly a wonder drug. It prevents up to 50 percent of heart attacks and strokes. There are also data that it offers some protection against several cancers, and possibly even Alzheimer's disease. About 162 mg, or two baby aspirin, seems to be the most appropriate dose for prevention, but 81 mg might be best for women.

10. **Take a multivitamin**. We recommend you get your vitamins from a variety of foods, especially fruits and vegetables. However, nutrition experts recommend a multivitamin daily for insurance. Take

those that have 100 percent of B3, B6, B12, folic acid, selenium, and vitamin D, but no excess of vitamin A and no more than 200 IU of vitamin E. A recent study showed that high doses of supplements can actually be harmful.

Enjoy your extra twenty QUALITY years!

## APPENDIX: RECIPES FOR A LONG AND HEALTHY LIFE

We have the good fortune to include in this book several excellent and simple recipes from *Cooking with Heart* by Richard Collins, MD, "The Cooking Cardiologist." Besides being a preeminent cardiologist, Dr. Collins is an expert chef with a passion for food, its presentation, and, of course, heart-healthy concepts.

Recipes reprinted with permission from *Cooking with Heart* by Richard Collins, MD (South Denver Heart Center; ISBN: 0-9778058-0-8). For more information or to order a copy of *Cooking with Heart*, please visit www.southdenver.com.

## VERY BERRY SALAD

¼ cup fresh orange juice

2 Tbsp. balsamic vinegar

1 Tbsp. firmly packed brown sugar

⅛ tsp. allspice

⅛ tsp. black pepper

3 cups fresh strawberries, halved

1 cup fresh raspberries

1 cup fresh blackberries

½ cup toasted walnuts

2 cups arugula

In a large bowl, whisk orange juice, vinegar, brown sugar, pepper, and allspice. Add the fruit and toss to coat. To serve, place a bed of arugula on a plate and top with the berry mixture. Garnish with additional berries and walnuts.

PREPARATION: EASY

NUMBER OF SERVINGS: 4

CARDIOLOGIST'S NOTE

Recent federal guidelines not only advise you to eat 2 cups of fruit per day, but also 2 ½ cups of vegetables per day. This new recommendation language is much clearer than the "serving size" language used in previous recommendations. The simple fact is that in America, fruit and fiber are eaten for breakfast only, and the rest of the day, Americans eat mostly meat and potatoes. Here is a salad recipe that has succulent fruit flavors and can be served with lunch or dinner. This salad is ideal in spring and summer when fresh berries are at their peak. Add grilled shrimp or a chicken breast for protein.

Nutrition information does not include shrimp or chicken breast.

NUTRITION INFORMATION

Serving Size: ¼ of recipe (232g)

*Amount per serving*

Calories 190   Calories from Fat 87

| | % Daily Value* |
|---|---|
| Total Fat 11g | 16% |
| Saturated Fat 1g | 5% |
| Cholesterol 0mg | 0% |
| Sodium 6mg | 0% |
| Total Carbohydrate 24g | 8% |
| Dietary Fiber 8g | 31% |
| Sugars 15g | |
| Protein 4g | |

| | |
|---|---|
| Vitamin A 8% | Vitamin C 149% |
| Calcium 7% | Iron 9% |

*Percent Daily Values are based on a 2,000 calorie diet.

# WALNUT ORANGE SPINACH SALAD

1 large garlic clove, minced

2 Tbsp. fresh lemon juice

2 Tbsp. red wine vinegar

1 Tbsp. honey

1 Tbsp. Italian parsley, chopped

⅛ tsp. black pepper

¼ cup fresh orange juice

2 Tbsp. walnut oil

8 cups crisp fresh spinach, washed

⅓ cup roasted walnuts

Place garlic, lemon juice, vinegar, honey, parsley, black pepper, orange juice, and oil in a bowl. Whisk until smooth. Toss with spinach and roasted walnuts. For variety, add sliced fresh pears to the salad.

PREPARATION: EASY
NUMBER OF SERVINGS: 8

CARDIOLOGIST'S NOTE

Dr. Richard Collins's philosophy: never buy food that can be stored in your kitchen for months. The only exceptions are wine and my grandmother's cellar-stored jar of peaches! Almost everyone has a salad dressing in their refrigerator door that has been there since last Thanksgiving or earlier. There is nothing better than salad dressing made from fresh, whole ingredients. In this recipe, the combination of roasted walnuts and walnut oil produces an intense flavor. Whether you use sesame seed, almond, or walnut oil, your next salad will have guests asking for more. Remember, a small amount of roasted nuts combined with nut oil of the same variety will increase flavor without adding extra fats. Say good-bye to cupfuls of oil, and enjoy the essence!

## NUTRITION INFORMATION

Serving Size: ⅛ of recipe (54g)

*Amount per serving*

Calories 82   Calories from Fat 54

| | % Daily Value* |
|---|---|
| Total Fat 7g | 10% |
| Saturated Fat 1g | 4% |
| Cholesterol 0mg | 0% |
| Sodium 24mg | 1% |
| Total Carbohydrate 5g | 2% |
| Dietary Fiber 1g | 5% |
| Sugars 3g | |
| Protein 2g | |

| | |
|---|---|
| Vitamin A 41% | Vitamin C 25% |
| Calcium 4% | Iron 6% |

*Percent Daily Values are based on a 2,000 calorie diet.

## MANGO GAZPACHO

1 mango, peeled and chopped
1 16-oz. can mango puree juice
1 bunch green onions, chopped
1 red bell pepper, chopped
1 yellow bell pepper, chopped
2 Tbsp. chopped cilantro
¼ cup rice vinegar
Juice of 1 lime
8 green bell peppers, chilled
1 jalapeño, chopped
Salt and black pepper to taste

Garnish:
1 cucumber, seeded
2 Tbsp. rice vinegar
Cilantro leaves

Combine all ingredients, except the garnish, in a large bowl. Mix well. For the garnish, slice cucumber into wedges. Lightly drizzle with rice vinegar. Serve gazpacho chilled with garnishes.

PREPARATION: EASY
NUMBER OF SERVINGS: 4

CARDIOLOGIST'S NOTE

Originating from the Andalusia region of Spain, this chilled soup is a summertime favorite. Traditional gazpacho is made with vinegar and tomatoes and other fresh garden vegetables, such as bell peppers, onions, cucumber, and garlic. The Americanized version has the southwest flavor found in the cilantro and lime combination.

This recipe adds a tangy new twist to the traditional version by using fresh mangos and prepared mango puree. Best of all, this chilled soup is loaded with vitamin C and colorful antioxidants. Serve in chilled, hollowed-out green bell peppers or martini glasses.

### NUTRITION INFORMATION

Serving Size: ¼ of recipe (462g)

*Amount per serving*

Calories 208    Calories from Fat 7

| | % Daily Value* |
|---|---|
| Total Fat 1g | 1% |
| Saturated Fat 0g | 1% |
| Cholesterol 0mg | 0% |
| Sodium 23mg | 1% |
| Total Carbohydrate 52g | 17% |
| Dietary Fiber 8g | 32% |
| Sugars 31g | |
| Protein 4g | |

| | |
|---|---|
| Vitamin A 82% | Vitamin C 491% |
| Calcium 7% | Iron 13% |

*Percent Daily Values are based on a 2,000 calorie diet.

## HUMMUS VEGGIE WRAP

2 fat-free 10-inch tortillas

4 Tbsp. softened fat-free cream cheese

4 Tbsp. pureed garbanzo beans (a.k.a. hummus)

1 small tomato, chopped

1 green onion, chopped

½ cup shredded leaf lettuce

2 Tbsp. fresh Italian parsley

2 Tbsp. salsa of choice

Spread the cream cheese over one tortilla, placing the second tortilla on top of the cream cheese. Spread the hummus on top of the second tortilla. Sprinkle with the chopped tomatoes, onions, lettuce, parsley, and salsa. Roll up tortilla and wrap tightly with plastic wrap. Chill to firm up the cream cheese. Slice in half, making two 5-inch wraps. Remove plastic and serve.

PREPARATION: EASY
NUMBER OF SERVINGS: 2

CARDIOLOGIST'S NOTE

These wraps are easy to make for a quick and tasty lunch. Try various salsas, from traditional tomato to mango or pineapple.

NUTRITION INFORMATION

Serving Size: ½ of recipe (178g)

*Amount per serving*

Calories 287    Calories from Fat 36

|  | % Daily Value* |
|---|---|
| Total Fat 4g | 6% |
| Saturated Fat 1g | 5% |
| Cholesterol 5mg | 2% |
| Sodium 937mg | 39% |
| Total Carbohydrate 47g | 16% |
| Dietary Fiber 6g | 23% |
| Sugars 3g | |
| Protein 17g | |

| Vitamin A 32% | Vitamin C 43% |
|---|---|
| Calcium 4% | Iron 8% |

*Percent Daily Values are based on a 2,000 calorie diet.

## ROASTED FENNEL AND ONIONS

Canola oil cooking spray
3 large sweet Vidalia onions, peeled and cut into wedges
2 fennel bulbs, cut into wedges, fronds reserved for garnish
2 Tbsp. balsamic vinegar
Ground black pepper to taste
1 Tbsp. brown sugar

Preheat oven to 400°. In a medium-sized roasting pan, coated lightly with canola oil, place onions and fennel. Drizzle the balsamic vinegar over the vegetables and toss to coat. Sprinkle black pepper and brown sugar over the top of the vegetables. Bake for one hour total, covered for 45 minutes of that hour. Check periodically and toss the vegetables to roast evenly. Remove when vegetables are tender. Finely chop half of the fennel bulb fronds. Garnish with whole and chopped fronds.

PREPARATION: EASY
NUMBER OF SERVINGS: 4

CARDIOLOGIST'S NOTE
The flavors of anise and onions are marvelous when roasted. The tartness of the balsamic vinegar is offset with the sweet brown sugar. This side dish is delicious and easy to make.

NUTRITION INFORMATION
Serving Size: ¼ of recipe (240g)

*Amount per serving*
Calories 93    Calories from Fat 3

|  | % Daily Value* |
|---|---|
| Total Fat 0g | 1% |
| Saturated Fat 0g | 0% |
| Cholesterol 0mg | 0% |
| Sodium 66mg | 3% |
| Total Carbohydrate 22g | 7% |
| Dietary Fiber 6g | 23% |
| Sugars 11g | |
| Protein 3g | |

| Vitamin A 3% | Vitamin C 35% |
|---|---|
| Calcium 8% | Iron 7% |

*Percent Daily Values are based on a 2,000 calorie diet.

# SWEET POTATO FRIES, A.K.A. "SWEETIES"

2 large sweet potatoes, washed and peeled
Salt to taste (optional)
Oil cooking spray
Parchment paper

Preheat oven to 400°. Cut potatoes lengthwise into finger-like pieces or use a French fry cutter. Line a baking sheet with parchment paper and lightly spray with cooking oil. Arrange potatoes in a single layer, not touching. Lightly spray the potatoes with cooking oil. Sprinkle with salt. Bake until golden brown, about 25 minutes. Turn once and adjust baking time as the potatoes brown.

PREPARATION: EASY
NUMBER OF SERVINGS: 2

CARDIOLOGIST'S NOTE

Contrary to popular belief, the majority of calories in French fries actually comes from the fat, not the carbohydrates. Sweet potatoes, even though "sweeter" in taste than white or red potatoes, have approximately the same number of carbohydrates per ounce. These fries are baked, which spares you more than 50 percent of the calories found in regular deep-fried fries.

NUTRITION INFORMATION

Serving Size: ½ of recipe (130g)

*Amount per serving*

Calories 136    Calories from Fat 3

|  | % Daily Value* |
|---|---|
| Total Fat 0g | 1% |
| Saturated Fat 0g | 0% |
| Cholesterol 0mg | 0% |
| Sodium 17mg | 1% |
| Total Carbohydrate 32g | 11% |
| Dietary Fiber 4g | 16% |
| Sugars 7g | |
| Protein 2g | |

| Vitamin A 522% | Vitamin C 49% |
|---|---|
| Calcium 3% | Iron 4% |

*Percent Daily Values are based on a 2,000 calorie diet.

## CHICKEN PENNE PRIMAVERA

8 oz. penne pasta
3 Tbsp. minced garlic
½ cup fat-free cream cheese
½ cup fat-free milk
¼ cup Parmesan cheese
Salt, to taste
2 boneless, skinless chicken breasts, cut into bite-sized pieces
1 4-oz. can quartered artichokes in water, cut into bite-sized pieces
1 4-oz. can sliced black olives, drained
6 asparagus spears, cut into bite-sized pieces
5 Tbsp. sun-dried tomatoes, chopped

In a large pot, boil water and add penne. Cook penne for 10 minutes and drain. Set aside. In a large skillet, sauté garlic and add chicken pieces until cooked. Remove chicken and set aside. In the same skillet on medium-low heat, melt cream cheese, milk, Parmesan and salt until smooth and creamy. Add chicken, artichokes, black olives, asparagus, sun-dried tomatoes, and penne. Continue cooking on medium-low heat for 15 minutes, until asparagus is cooked to desired tenderness.

PREPARATION: INTERMEDIATE
NUMBER OF SERVINGS: 4

NUTRITION INFORMATION
Serving Size: ¼ of recipe (199g)

*Amount per serving*
Calories 371    Calories from Fat 39

| | % Daily Value* |
|---|---|
| Total Fat 4g | 7% |
| Saturated Fat 2g | 8% |
| Cholesterol 27mg | 9% |
| Sodium 760mg | 32% |
| Total Carbohydrate 56g | 19% |
| Dietary Fiber 6g | 23% |
| Sugars 6g | |
| Protein 26g | |

| | |
|---|---|
| Vitamin A 10% | Vitamin C 13% |
| Calcium 20% | Iron 20% |

*Percent Daily Values are based on a 2,000 calorie diet.

## HERB-GRILLED TROUT

3 trout fillets (4-6 oz. each)

1 lemon, sliced

1 sprig fresh dill

1 sprig thyme

4–5 chives, uncut

Salt and pepper, to taste

Twine

Oil

With the skin on the whole fillet, open the trout. Place herbs divided equally among the fish fillets. Add salt and pepper, to taste. Close the fillet and place lemon slices on the outside. Tie with moistened twine. Place trout skin-side down on a medium-hot grill that has been rubbed with oil to prevent sticking. Turn once and grill until fish fillets are cooked. Mist with water to help steam the fish and keep the twine moist while grilling. Serve with roasted vegetables. Wonderful!

PREPARATION: EASY
NUMBER OF SERVINGS: 3

CARDIOLOGIST'S NOTE

This recipe is the easiest trout recipe around and will have your family and guests asking for more. It uses fresh trout fillets and herbs, placed in a pocket in the middle of the fillet. Herbs and a hot grill do not mix, unless the herbs are well inside the food item. This cooking process steams the herbs into the fish on the inside. Serve the trout with a rich glass of white wine, such as a chilled chardonnay.

NUTRITION INFORMATION

Serving Size: ⅓ of recipe (149g)

*Amount per serving*

Calories 175   Calories from Fat 67

|  | % Daily Value* |
|---|---|
| Total Fat 8g | 12% |
| Saturated Fat 1g | 7% |
| Cholesterol 66mg | 22% |
| Sodium 60mg | 3% |
| Total Carbohydrate 4g | 1% |
| Dietary Fiber 2g | 7% |
| Sugars 1g | |
| Protein 24g | |

| Vitamin A 2% | Vitamin C 47% |
|---|---|
| Calcium 7% | Iron 11% |

*Percent Daily Values are based on a 2,000 calorie diet.

## CHICKEN WITH CHINESE VEGETABLE STIR-FRY

4 skinless, boneless chicken breasts, sliced into thin pieces
  OR 8.5 oz. vegetarian chicken substitute
1 tsp. salt substitute
½ egg white, slightly beaten
2 tsp. cornstarch paste (1 tsp. cornstarch and 2 tsp. water)
3 Tbsp. tea oil or canola oil
1 tsp. fresh ginger, chopped
2 garlic cloves, chopped
1 scallion, cut into short sections
1 4-oz. can sliced bamboo shoots, drained
4 oz. snow peas
8 small shiitake mushrooms, chopped
1 tsp. light brown sugar
1 Tbsp. reduced-sodium soy sauce
1 Tbsp. rice wine or sherry

Prepare the chicken and place in a glass bowl with salt, egg white, and cornstarch paste. Mix. Prepare all vegetables and heat the wok, adding oil to coat the sides. Add the chicken and stir-fry for 1 minute. Remove with slotted spoon and keep warm. Add the ginger, garlic, and scallions. Toss for a few seconds, and then add remaining vegetables. Toss and mix for approximately 1–2 minutes, adding the brown sugar and chicken. Blend, then add the soy sauce and rice wine. Additional cornstarch paste may be added to thicken the sauce. Serve over Chinese noodles or whole-grain rice.

PREPARATION: EASY
NUMBER OF SERVINGS: 4

CARDIOLOGIST'S NOTE
The art of stir-frying is simple, yet requires a few pointers to ensure a great result. The success is in the use of a good quality wok and high heat. Start by heating the wok over high heat. Use a healthy quantity of oil; tea oil is the best, but

canola oil will suffice. Add just enough oil to lightly coat the sides by swirling and tilting the wok. The oil should be hot. Add the ingredients in the order specified. First add the aromatics—garlic, ginger, and scallions. Toss for only a few seconds, adding the main ingredients, such as dense vegetables or meat, next. Keep the ingredients moving with a wok scoop. Remember, there is a tendency to overcook vegetables. Serve directly from the wok.

## NUTRITION INFORMATION

Serving Size: ¼ of recipe (158g)

*Amount per serving*

Calories 200    Calories from Fat 73

|  | % Daily Value* |
|---|---|
| Total Fat 8g | 13% |
| Saturated Fat 1g | 6% |
| Cholesterol 41mg | 14% |
| Sodium 210mg | 9% |
| Total Carbohydrate 12g | 4% |
| Dietary Fiber 2g | 9% |
| Sugars 3g | |
| Protein 19g | |

| | |
|---|---|
| Vitamin A 1% | Vitamin C 5% |
| Calcium 2% | Iron 6% |

*Percent Daily Values are based on a 2,000 calorie diet.

## MICROWAVE HERB TROUT

10 oz. frozen trout fillets
1 Tbsp. scallions, finely chopped
3 Tbsp. mushrooms, finely chopped
2 Tbsp. green bell pepper, finely chopped
2 Tbsp. celery, finely chopped
1 tsp. oregano
1 tsp. basil
1 tsp. paprika
1 tsp. lemon juice
2 Tbsp. breadcrumbs
1 ½ Tbsp. plant-sterol margarine, melted

Remove trout fillets from the freezer. Cover and cook 4 minutes in the microwave on high. Skin the trout and separate into pieces. Layer in a casserole dish and cover with scallions, mushrooms, green bell pepper, and celery. Sprinkle with oregano, basil, and paprika, to taste. Add lemon juice and breadcrumbs. Drizzle melted margarine over the top and cover. Cook on high for approximately 1–2 minutes. (Be careful not to overcook as it will become too dry.)

PREPARATION: EASY
NUMBER OF SERVINGS: 2

NUTRITION INFORMATION
Serving Size: ½ of recipe (159g)

*Amount per serving*
Calories 229  Calories from Fat 102

|  | % Daily Value* |
|---|---|
| Total Fat 11g | 17% |
| Saturated Fat 2g | 8% |
| Cholesterol 67mg | 22% |
| Sodium 183mg | 8% |
| Total Carbohydrate 6g | 2% |
| Dietary Fiber 1g | 3% |
| Sugars 1g | |
| Protein 24g | |

| | |
|---|---|
| Vitamin A 3% | Vitamin C 20% |
| Calcium 10% | Iron 8% |

*Percent Daily Values are based on a 2,000 calorie diet.

# TUSCAN TUNA AND CANNELLINI BEANS

⅓ cup orange juice

1 onion, chopped

⅔ cup dry vermouth or dry white wine

¼ cup white wine vinegar

1 lb. fresh tuna steaks, cut into 1-inch cubes

4 cups cooked cannellini beans or canned beans, rinsed and drained

2 tomatoes, coarsely chopped

¼ cup fresh basil, chopped

½ tsp. black pepper

2 Tbsp. orange zest, grated

1 Tbsp. chives, chopped

In a large nonstick frying pan over medium-high heat, heat the orange juice. Add the onion and sauté until softened, about 5 minutes. Add the vermouth or wine and vinegar and continue to sauté for 2 minutes. Reduce heat to medium, and stir in the fish, beans, tomatoes, basil, pepper, and half the orange zest. Cover and cook until the fish is opaque throughout, about 7–9 minutes. To serve, divide among individual plates. Sprinkle with the chives and remaining orange zest.

PREPARATION: INTERMEDIATE

NUMBER OF SERVINGS: 6

CARDIOLOGIST'S NOTE

Tuna and white beans, or tonno e fagioli, is a favorite in Tuscan kitchens, enjoyed for the way the creamy legumes complement the firm-textured fish. Here, orange juice and zest add a tangy, fruity flavor that highlights both featured ingredients.

NUTRITION INFORMATION

Serving Size: 1/6 of recipe (338g)

*Amount per serving*

Calories 341    Calories from Fat 14

| | % Daily Value* |
|---|---|
| Total Fat 1g | 2% |
| Saturated Fat 0g | 2% |
| Cholesterol 34mg | 11% |
| Sodium 44mg | 2% |
| Total Carbohydrate 45g | 15% |
| Dietary Fiber 9g | 38% |
| Sugars 11g | |
| Protein 31g | |

| | |
|---|---|
| Vitamin A 8% | Vitamin C 34% |
| Calcium 15% | Iron 34% |

*Percent Daily Values are based on a 2,000 calorie diet.

## ROASTED MAPLE SALMON

1 cup reduced-sodium soy sauce
1 cup maple syrup
4 4-oz. Pacific Northwest salmon fillets

For the marinade, place the soy sauce and the maple syrup in a plastic zip-top bag. Add the salmon fillets. Marinate for four hours or overnight in the refrigerator.

Preheat oven to 350°. On a large baking sheet covered with aluminum foil, place the fillets skin-side down. Discard excess marinade. Bake for approximately 10–15 minutes, until salmon is fully cooked. Serve with mashed sweet potatoes and steamed vegetables.

PREPARATION: EASY
NUMBER OF SERVINGS: 4

CARDIOLOGIST'S NOTE

This is my favorite salmon recipe, and it's "soy" easy to make. This is truly a crowd-pleaser, with the sweetness of the maple sugar and the saltiness of soy sauce balancing each other.

NUTRITION INFORMATION

Serving Size: ¼ of recipe (170g)

*Amount per serving*

Calories 265   Calories from Fat 54

|  | % Daily Value* |
|---|---|
| Total Fat 6g | 9% |
| Saturated Fat 1g | 6% |
| Cholesterol 45mg | 15% |
| Sodium 1,112mg | 46% |
| Total Carbohydrate 29g | 10% |
| Dietary Fiber 0g | 1% |
| Sugars 28g | |
| Protein 23g | |

| | |
|---|---|
| Vitamin A 2% | Vitamin C 2% |
| Calcium 7% | Iron 9% |

*Percent Daily Values are based on a 2,000 calorie diet.

## SALMON IN A POUCH

1 lb. Alaskan salmon fillet, cut into 2x2-inch squares
Splash of vermouth (optional)
2 cups assorted vegetables—green onions, diced carrots, new potatoes,
zucchini, etc.
¼ cup fresh dill, chopped
¼ cup fresh tarragon, chopped
¼ cup fresh thyme, chopped
4 Tbsp. vegetable broth or water
4 14x14-inch square parchment sheets
Twine

If desired, sprinkle vermouth over salmon 30 minutes before preparation. Place all ingredients, divided equally, onto four parchment paper sheets. Add one tablespoon vegetable broth to each serving. Bring edges up to tie into a pouch. Place in microwave on high for 5–7 minutes. If microwaving four servings at a time, increase time appropriately. Or bake pouches in oven at 375° for 15 minutes. Serve on plates with scissors handy. Open pouches and garnish with extra herbs.

PREPARATION: EASY
NUMBER OF SERVINGS: 4

NUTRITION INFORMATION

Serving Size: ¼ of recipe (218g)

*Amount per serving*

Calories 212   Calories from Fat 80

| | % Daily Value* |
|---|---|
| Total Fat 9g | 14% |
| Saturated Fat 2g | 10% |
| Cholesterol 58mg | 19% |
| Sodium 72mg | 3% |
| Total Carbohydrate 7g | 2% |
| Dietary Fiber 2g | 9% |
| Sugars 3g | |
| Protein 26g | |

| | |
|---|---|
| Vitamin A 95% | Vitamin C 24% |
| Calcium 3% | Iron 6% |

*Percent Daily Values are based on a 2,000 calorie diet.

## POLENTA WITH SUN-DRIED TOMATO PESTO

For the polenta:
4 cups vegetable broth
2 cups water
2 cups cornmeal
2 Tbsp. plant-sterol margarine
½ tsp. garlic powder
Dash of freshly ground nutmeg
Salt and pepper to taste

For the tomato pesto sauce:
1 cup softened sun-dried tomatoes
2 cloves garlic, chopped
½ cup balsamic vinegar
1 cup fresh basil, chopped
½ cup fresh Italian parsley, chopped
2 large tomatoes, peeled and seeded

For garnish:
¼ cup shaved Parmesan cheese

In a large saucepan, add the vegetable broth and water and bring to a boil. Gradually stir in the cornmeal. Reduce heat. Stir frequently to thicken and avoid a lumpy polenta. Add the margarine, garlic, and nutmeg. Add salt and pepper to taste. Continue cooking until thickened. Cool and spread on an oil-sprayed 10x15-inch baking sheet. Refrigerate. When firm, cut into various shapes using a cookie cutter. Three-inch-size hearts are perfect for this heart-healthy polenta. Place on heated grill. Grill for 5–10 minutes to sear the polenta. For the pesto, place all ingredients into a blender or small food processor and process until smooth. Before serving, warm pesto sauce and spoon 1–2 tablespoons over each serving of polenta. Add a shaving of Parmesan cheese.

PREPARATION: INTERMEDIATE

NUMBER OF SERVINGS: 10

CARDIOLOGIST'S NOTE

Polenta (poh-LEHN-tah) is an Italian dish derived from cornmeal. It can be served soft, as a mush, or firm, grill-roasted. Usually it is thickened with cheese, Parmesan or gorgonzola, and butter. The secret to smooth polenta is in the attention to stirring on the stovetop. Polenta is usually accompanied with a tomato topping. It can be served as a side dish, first course, or even breakfast—like grits, a southern American corn dish.

## NUTRITION INFORMATION

Serving Size: 1/10 of recipe (91g)

*Amount per serving*

Calories 149  Calories from Fat 32

| | % Daily Value* |
|---|---|
| Total Fat 4g | 6% |
| Saturated Fat 1g | 4% |
| Cholesterol 1mg | 0% |
| Sodium 367mg | 15% |
| Total Carbohydrate 27g | 9% |
| Dietary Fiber 3g | 13% |
| Sugars 3g | |
| Protein 4g | |

| | |
|---|---|
| Vitamin A 14% | Vitamin C 28% |
| Calcium 5% | Iron 11% |

*Percent Daily Values are based on a 2,000 calorie diet.

# LOW-FAT "EGG SAUSAGE" BREAKFAST SANDWICH

1 whole-wheat English muffin
¼ cup egg substitute
1 breakfast sausage substitute patty
1 slice fat-free American cheese
1 Tbsp. salsa (optional)
Chopped cilantro for garnish (optional)

Toast the muffin. In a 3-inch ramekin, lightly mist with cooking spray to coat sides to prevent sticking. Place the sausage patty in bottom of ramekin. Pour egg substitute over the sausage to cover. Microwave on high for 2 minutes, 22 seconds , or until egg substitute is firm. Remove from microwave.

Caution: ramekin may be hot.

Place cooked egg substitute and sausage on English muffin and cover with a slice of cheese. Top with the other half of the toasted muffin.

For a southwest flavor, add salsa and chopped cilantro.

PREPARATION: EASY
NUMBER OF SERVINGS: 1

CARDIOLOGIST'S NOTE
America is the only place where it takes one calorie to roll down your car window to get a 700-calorie breakfast. A conventional fast-food breakfast sandwich has about 29 grams of fat and twice the number of calories as this low-fat egg sausage sandwich. This recipe is fast to prepare and tastes just like the drive-up window meal without the nitrites, excess salt, cholesterol and fat. All of the ingredients are available nationally in standard grocery stores.

## NUTRITION INFORMATION
Serving Size: 1 (66g)

*Amount per serving*

Calories 268   Calories from Fat 39

|  | % Daily Value* |
|---|---|
| Total Fat 4g | 7% |
| Saturated Fat 1g | 4% |
| Cholesterol 2mg | 1% |
| Sodium 1,049mg | 44% |
| Total Carbohydrate 33g | 11% |
| Dietary Fiber 6g | 26% |
| Sugars 6g | |
| Protein 25g | |

| | |
|---|---|
| Vitamin A 0% | Vitamin C 0% |
| Calcium 17% | Iron 9% |

*Percent Daily Values are based on a 2,000 calorie diet.

# NOTES

## Preface

M. Reeves and A. Rafferty, "Healthy Lifestyle Characteristics Among Adults in the U.S., 2000," *Archives of Internal Medicine* 165 (25 April 2005), 854–857.

S. Chiuve et al., "Healthy Lifestyle Factors in the Primary Prevention of CHD Among Men: Benefits Among Users and Nonusers of Lipid-Lowering and Anti-hypertensive Medications," *Circulation* 114 (11 July 2006), 160–167.

## Chapter 1
## A Great Time to Live a Long Life

S. Jay Olshansky and Bruce A. Carnes, *The Quest for Immortality: Science at the Frontiers of Aging* (New York: W. W. Norton, 2001).

*Health, United States, 2005 with Chartbook on Trends in the Health of Americans*, (Hyattsville, Md.: CDC National Center for Health Statistics Press, 2005), Table 26.

Joseph C. G. Kennedy, "Preliminary Report of the Eighth Census," U.S. Census Bureau, Washington, D.C., 1862.

Donna L. Hoyert et al., "Deaths, Final Data for 2003," *National Vital Statistics Reports* 54, no. 13 (April 2006).

Scott M. Grundy, "Age as a Risk Factor: You Are as Old as Your Arteries," *The American Journal of Cardiology* 83 (15 May 1999), 1455–1457.

Salim Yusuf et al., "Effect of Potentially Modifiable Risk Factors Associated with

Myocardial Infarction in 52 Countries (the INTERHEART Study): Case-Control Study," *Lancet* 364 (11 September 2004), 937–952.

Richard Doll and Richard Peto, "The Causes of Cancer: Quantitative Estimates of Avoidable Risks of Cancer in the United States Today," *Journal of the National Cancer Institute* 66 (June 1981), 1191–1308.

## Chapter 2
## Understanding the Biggest Threats to Your Longevity

Erling Falk, Prediman K. Shah, and Valentin Fuster, "Coronary Plaque Disruption," *Circulation* 92 (August 1995), 657–671.

D. Larry Sparks et al., "Link Between Heart Disease, Cholesterol, and Alzheimer's Disease: A Review," *Microscopy Research and Technique* 50 (August 2000), 287–290.

R. G. DePalma et al., "Regression of Atherosclerotic Plaques in Rhesus Monkeys: Angiographic, Morphologic, and Angiochemical Changes," *Archives of Surgery* 115 (November 1980), 1268–1278.

M. R. Malinow, "Atherosclerosis: Regression in Nonhuman Primates," *Circulation Research* 46 (March 1980), 311–320.

Steven E. Nissen et al., "Effect of Intensive Compared with Moderate Lipid-Lowering Therapy on Progression of Coronary Atherosclerosis: A Randomized Controlled Trial," *JAMA: The Journal of the American Medical Association* 291 (3 March 2004), 1071–1080.

Steven E. Nissen et al., "Effect of Very High-Intensity Statin Therapy on Regression of Coronary Atherosclerosis: The ASTEROID Trial," *JAMA: The Journal of the American Medical Association* 295 (5 April 2006), 1556–1565.

G. A. Ramirez-Granillo, "Meta-analysis of the Studies Assessing Temporal Changes in Coronary Plaque Volume Using Intravascular Ultrasound," *The American Journal of Cardiology* 99 (1 January 2007), 5–10.

Ilke Sipahi et al., "Effects of Normal, Pre-Hypertensive, and Hypertensive Blood Pressure Levels on Progression of Coronary Atherosclerosis," *Journal of the American College of Cardiology* 48 (August 2006), 833–838.

S. Lewington et al. for the Prospective Studies Collaboration, "Age-Specific Reference of Usual Blood Pressure to Vascular Mortality: A Meta-analysis of Individual Data for One Million Adults in 61 Prospective Studies," *Lancet* 360 (14 December 2002), 1903–1913.

R. S. Vasan et al., "Impact of High-Normal Blood Pressure on the Risk of Cardio-vascular Disease," *New England Journal of Medicine* 345 (1 November 2001), 1291–1296.

William F. Enos, Robert H. Holmes, and James Beyer, "Coronary Disease Among United States Soldiers Killed in Action in Korea," *JAMA: The Journal of the American Medical Association* 152 (18 July 1953), 1090–1093.

The Pathobiological Determinants of Atherosclerosis in Youth (PDAY) Research Group, "Relationship of Atherosclerosis in Young Men to Serum Lipoprotein Cholesterol Concentrations and Smoking," *JAMA: The Journal of the American Medical Association* 264 (19 December 1990), 3018–3024.

Gerald S. Berenson et al., "Association Between Multiple Cardiovascular Risk Factors and Atherosclerosis in Children and Young Adults," *New England Journal of Medicine* 338 (4 June 1998), 1650–1656.

L. A. G. Ries et al., *SEER Cancer Statistics Review, 1975–2003*, National Cancer Institute, Bethesda, Md., http://seer.cancer.gov/csr/1975_2003/, 2006.

Richard Doll and Richard Peto, "The Causes of Cancer: Quantitative Estimates of Avoidable Risks of Cancer in the United States Today," *Journal of the National Cancer Institute* 66 (June 1981), 1191–1308.

Clyde W. Yancy et al., "Discovering the Full Spectrum of Cardiovascular Disease: Minority Health Summit 2003," *Circulation* 111 (March 2005), 1339–1349.

C. Nielson, T. Lange, and N. Hadjokas, "Blood Glucose and Coronary Artery Disease in Nondiabetic Patients," *Diabetes Care* 5 (29 May 2006), 998–1001.

Joanne Davidson, "Star Lights Up Alzheimer's Luncheon," *Denver Post*, 1 December 2005, F1.

D. Larry Sparks et al., "Link Between Heart Disease, Cholesterol, and Alzheimer's Disease: A Review," *Microscopy Research and Technique* 50 (August 2000), 287–290.

D. Larry Sparks et al., "Atorvastatin for the Treatment of Mild to Moderate Alzheimer's Disease," *Archives of Neurology* 62 (May 2005), 753–757.

Alex E. Roher et al., "Circle of Willis Atherosclerosis Is a Risk Factor for Sporadic Alzheimer's Disease," *Arteriosclerosis, Thrombosis, and Vascular Biology* 23 (November 2003), 2055–2062.

Costantino Iadecola, "Atherosclerosis and Neurodegeneration: Unexpected Conspirators in Alzheimer's Dementia," *Arteriosclerosis, Thrombosis, and Vascular Biology* 23 (November 2003), 1951–1953.

## Chapter 3
## Your Personal Risk Profile

O. Turpeinen, "Effect of Cholesterol-Lowering Diet on Mortality from Coronary Artery Disease and Other Causes," *Circulation* 59 (January 1979), 1–7.

W. M. Verschuren et al., "Serum Total Cholesterol and Long-Term Coronary Heart Disease Mortality in Different Cultures: Twenty-Five Year Follow-Up of the Seven Country Study," *JAMA: The Journal of the American Medical Association* 274 (12 July 1995), 131–136.

E. Vartiainen et al., "Changes in Risk Factors Explain Changes in Mortality from Ischemic Heart Disease in Finland," *British Medical Journal* 309 (2 July 1994), 23–27.

T. Laatikainen et al., "Explaining the Decline in Coronary Heart Disease Mortality in Finland Between 1982 and 1997," *American Journal of Epidemiology* 162 (15 April 2005), 764–773.

J. C. LaRosa et al., "The Cholesterol Facts: A Summary of the Evidence Relating Dietary Fats, Serum Cholesterol, and Coronary Heart Disease. A Joint Statement by the American Heart Association and the National Heart, Lung, and Blood Institute" *Circulation* 81 (May 1990), 1721–1733.

B. B. Dean et al., "Can Change in HDL-Cholesterol Reduce Cardiovascular Risk?" *American Heart Journal* 147 (June 2004), 966–976.

H. B. Rubins, "Triglycerides and Coronary Heart Disease: Implications of Recent Clinical Trials," *Journal of Cardiovascular Risk* 7 (October 2000), 339–345.

Ilene Springer, "'Against All Odds,' Dr. William Castelli: A Pioneer Speaks Out," Lifestyle Medicine Institute, http://www.chipusa.org/downloads/Section3_1316.pdf, accessed March 2007.

W. C. Roberts, "Atherosclerotic Risk Factors—Are There Ten or Is There Only One?" *The American Journal of Cardiology* 64 (1 September 1989), 552–554.

T. L. Robertson et al., "Epidemiologic Studies of Coronary Heart Disease and Stroke in Japanese Men Living in Japan, Hawaii, and California: Coronary Heart Disease Risk Factors in Japan and Hawaii," *The American Journal of Cardiology* 39 (February 1977), 244–249.

O. Turpeinen, "Effect of Cholesterol-Lowering Diet on Mortality from Coronary Heart Disease and Other Causes," *Circulation* 59 (January 1979), 1–7.

Julian Whitaker, *Reversing Heart Disease* (New York: Warner Books, 1985).

R. S. Vasan et al., "Impact of High-Normal Blood Pressure on the Risk of Cardiovascular Disease," *New England Journal of Medicine* 345 (1 November 2001), 1291–1297.

S. Lewington et al., "Age-Specific Relevance of Usual Blood Pressure to Vascular Mortality: A Meta-analysis of Individual Data for One Million Adults in 61 Prospective Studies," *Lancet* 360 (14 December 2002), 1903–1913.

Joint National Committee on Prevention, Detection, Evaluation, and Treatment of High Blood Pressure, "The Seventh Report of the Joint National Committee on Prevention, Detection, Evaluation, and Treatment of High Blood Pressure," *JAMA: The Journal of the American Medical Association* 289 (21 May 2003), 2561–2572.

Robert Ferrell, *The Dying President: Franklin D. Roosevelt, 1944–1945* (Columbia: University of Missouri Press, 1998).

M. Ezzati and A. Lopez, "Estimates of Global Mortality Attributable to Smoking in 2000," *Lancet* 362 (13 September 2003), 847–852.

Terry F. Pechacek and Stephen Babb, "How Acute and Reversible are the Cardio-vascular Risks of Secondhand Smoke?" *British Medical Journal* 328 (24 April 2004), 980–983.

R. P. Sargent, R. M. Shepard, and S. A. Glantz, "Reduced Incidence of Admissions for Myocardial Infarction Associated with Public Smoking Ban: Before and After Study," *British Medical Journal* 328 (24 April 2004), 977–980.

Carl Bartecchi et al., "Reduction in the Incidence of Acute Myocardial Infarction Associated with a Citywide Smoking Ordinance," *Circulation* 114 (3 October 2006), 1490–1496.

C. Iribarren et al., "Effect of Cigar Smoking on the Risk of Cardiovascular Disease, Chronic Obstructive Pulmonary Disease, and Cancer in Men," *New England Journal of Medicine* 340 (10 June 1999), 1773–1780.

R. Gupta et al. "Smokeless Tobacco and Cardiovascular Risk," *Archives of Internal Medicine* 164 (27 September 2004), 1845–1849.

B. H. Marcus et al., "The Efficacy of Exercise as an Aid for Smoking Cessation in Women: A Randomized Controlled Trial," *Archives of Internal Medicine* 159 (14 June 1999), 1229–1234.

R. E. Ratner, "An Update on the Diabetes Prevention Program," *Endocrine Practice,* 12, Supplement 1 (January–February 2006), 20–24.

S. Yusuf et al., "Effect of Potentially Modifiable Risk Factors Associated with Myocardial Infarction in 52 Countries (the INTERHEART Study): Case-Control Study," *Lancet* 364 (11–17 September 2004), 937–952.

Pekka Jousilahti et al., "Sex, Age, Cardiovascular Risk Factors, and Coronary Heart Disease: A Prospective Follow-Up Study of 14,786 Middle-Aged Men and Women in Finland," *Circulation* 99 (March 1999), 1165–1172.

American Heart Association, "Heart Disease and Stroke Statistics: 2004 Update," American Heart Association, Dallas, TX, 2003.

## Chapter 4
## Exercise: The Real Fountain of Youth

G. A. Kelley, K. S. Kelley, and Z. V. Tran, "Walking, Lipids, and Lipoproteins: A Meta-analysis of Randomized Controlled Trials," *Preventive Medicine* 38 (May 2004), 51–61.

William E. Kraus et al., "Effects of the Amount and Intensity of Exercise on Plasma Lipoproteins," *New England Journal of Medicine* 347 (7 November 2002), 1483–1492.

Mercedes R. Carnethon, Martha Gulati, and Philip Greenland, "Prevalence and Cardiovascular Disease Correlates of Low Cardiorespiratory Fitness in Adolescents and Adults," *JAMA: The Journal of the American Medical Association* 294 (21 December 2005), 2981–2988.

Timo A. Lakka et al., "Effect of Exercise Training on Plasma Levels of C-reactive Protein in Healthy Adults: The HERITAGE Family Study," *European Heart Journal* 26 (October 2005), 2018–2025.

American Psychological Association, "Exercise Helps Sustain Mental Activity as We Age and May Prevent Dementia-like Illness," press release, 11 August 2006.

Stanley J. Colcombe et al., "Cardiovascular Fitness, Cortical Plasticity, and Aging," *PNAS: Proceedings of the National Academy of Sciences of the United States of America* 101 (2 March 2004), 3316–3321.

Kristine Yaffe et al., "A Prospective Study of Physical Activity and Cognitive Decline in Elderly Women: Women Who Walk," *Archives of Internal Medicine* 161 (23 July 2001), 1703–1708.

Jerome L. Fleg et al., "Accelerated Longitudinal Decline of Aerobic Capacity in Healthy Older Adults," *Circulation* 112 (August 2005), 674–682.

T. Ogawa et al., "Effects of Aging, Sex, and Physical Training on Cardiovascular Responses to Exercise," *Circulation* 86 (August 1992), 494–503.

Rainer Hambrecht et al., "Percutaneous Coronary Angioplasty Compared with

Exercise Training in Patients with Stable Coronary Artery Disease: A Randomized Trial," *Circulation* 109 (23 March 2004), 1371–1378.

C. J. Lavie, R. V. Milani, and A. B. Littman, "Benefits of Cardiac Rehabilitation and Exercise Training in Secondary Coronary Prevention in the Elderly," *JACC: Journal of the American College of Cardiology* 22 (September 1993), 678–683.

D. Rothenbacher et al., "Lifetime Physical Activity Patterns and Risk of Coronary Heart Disease," *Heart* 92 (September 2006), 1319–1320.

A. W. Gardner and E. T. Poehlman, "Exercise Rehabilitation Programs for the Treatment of Claudication Pain: A Meta-analysis," *JAMA: The Journal of the American Medical Association* 274 (27 September 1995), 975–980.

Ming Wei et al., "Relationship Between Low Cardiorespiratory Fitness and Mortality in Normal-Weight, Overweight, and Obese Men," *JAMA: The Journal of the American Medical Association* 282 (27 October 1999), 1547–1553.

T. S. Church et al., "Cardiorespiratory Fitness and Body Mass Index as Predictors of Cardiovascular Disease Mortality Among Men with Diabetes," *Archives of Internal Medicine* 165 (10 October 2005), 2114–2120.

S. N. Blair et al., "Influences of Cardiorespiratory Fitness and Other Precursors on Cardiovascular Disease and All-Cause Mortality in Men and Women," *JAMA: The Journal of the American Medical Association* 276 (17 July 1996), 205–210.

R. R. Pate et al., "Physical Activity and Public Health: A Recommendation from the Centers for Disease Control and Prevention and the American College of Sports Medicine," *JAMA: The Journal of the American Medical Association* 273 (1 February 1995), 402–407.

L. H. Kushi et al., "American Cancer Society Guidelines on Nutrition and Physical Activity for Cancer Prevention: Reducing the Risk of Cancer with Healthy Food Choices and Physical Activity," *CA: A Cancer Journal for Clinicians* 56 (September–October 2006), 254–281.

Ralph S. Paffenbarger, Alvin L. Wing, and Robert T. Hyde, "Physical Activity as an Index of Heart Attack Risk in College Alumni," *American Journal of Epidemiology* 108 (September 1978), 161–175.

## Chapter 5
### Diet: Personal Choices with Huge Impacts

Bradley J. Willcox, D. Craig Willcox, and Makoto Suzuki, *The Okinawa Program:*

*How the World's Longest-Lived People Achieve Everlasting Health—And How You Can Too* (New York: Clarkson Potter, 2001).

Walter C. Willett, *Eat, Drink and Be Healthy: The Harvard Medical School Guide to Healthy Eating* (New York: Simon and Schuster, 2001).

"Health Department Proposes Two Changes to City's Health Code for Public Comment: First, to Phase Out Artificial Trans Fat in All Restaurants; Second, to Require Calorie Labeling in Some Restaurants," press release, NYC Department of Health and Mental Hygiene, 26 September 2006, http://www.nyc.gov/html/doh/html/pr2006/pr093-06.shtml.

Martijn B. Katan et al., "Efficacy and Safety of Plant Stanols and Sterols in the Management of Blood Cholesterol Levels," *Mayo Clinic Proceedings* 178 (August 2003), 965–978.

A. H. Lichtenstein and R. J. Deckelbaum, "AHA Science Advisory: Stanol/Sterol Ester-Containing Foods and Blood Cholesterol Levels: A Statement for Healthcare Professionals from the Nutrition Committee of the Council on Nutrition, Physical Activity, and Metabolism of the American Heart Association," *Circulation* 103 (27 February 2001), 1177–1179.

Reader's Digest Editors, *Foods That Harm, Foods That Heal* (New York: Readers Digest, 2004).

M. Covas et al., "The Effect of Polyphenols in Olive Oil on Heart Disease Risk Factors," *Annals of Internal Medicine* 145 (5 September 2006), 333–341.

Dario Giuglianoet al., "Effect of Diet on Inflammation," *Journal of the American College of Cardiology* 48 (15 August 2006), 677–685.

A. Basu et al., "Dietary Factors That Promote or Retard Inflammation," *Arteriosclerosis, Thrombosis, and Vascular Biology* 26 (May 2006), 995–1001.

M. Daviglus et al., "Fish Consumption and the 30-Year Risk of Fatal Myocardial Infarction," *New England Journal of Medicine* 336 (10 April 1997), 1046–1053.

F. B. Hu et al., "Fish and Omega-3 Fatty Acid Intake and Risk of Coronary Heart Disease in Women," *JAMA: The Journal of the American Medical Association* 287 (10 April 2002), 1815–1821.

C. Albert et al., "Blood Levels of Long-Chain Omega-3 Fatty Acids and the Risk of Sudden Death," *New England Journal of Medicine* 346 (11 April 2002), 1113–1118.

M. Morris et al., "Consumption of Fish and Omega-3 Fatty Acids and Risk of Incident Alzheimer's Disease," *Archives of Neurology* 60 (July 2003), 940–946.

J. G. Robinson and N. J. Stone, "Antiatherosclerotic and Antithrombotic Effects of Omega-3 Fatty Acids," *The American Journal of Cardiology* 99 (21 August 2006), 39i–49i.

Johanna M. Seddon et al., "Cigarette Smoking, Fish Consumption, Omega-3 Fatty Acid Intake, and Associations with Age-Related Macular Degeneration," *Archives of Ophthalmology* 124 (July 2006), 995–1001.

P. Kris-Etherton et al., "Omega-3 Fatty Acids and Cardiovascular Disease: New Recommendations from the American Heart Association," *Arteriosclerosis, Thrombosis, Vascular Biology* 23 (1 February 2003), 151–152.

Penny M. Kris-Etherton et al., "American Heart Association Scientific Statement: Fish Consumption, Fish Oil, Omega-3 Fatty Acids, and Cardiovascular Disease," *Circulation* 106 (19 November 2002), 2747–2757.

Institute of Medicine of the National Academies, "Seafood Choices: Balancing Benefits and Risks. Report of the Committee on Nutrient Relationships in Seafood: Selections to Balance Benefits and Risks," http://www.iom.edu/CMS/3788/23788/37679.aspx, accessed on October 2006.

D. Mozaffarian and E. Rimmm, "Fish Intake, Contaminants, and Human Health," *JAMA: The Journal of the American Medical Association* 296 (18 October 2006), 1885–1899.

G. Fraser et al., "A Possible Protective Effect of Nut Consumption on Risk of Coronary Heart Disease: The Adventist Health Study," *Archives of Internal Medicine* 152 (1 July 1992), 1416–1424.

Frank B. Hu et al., "Frequent Nut Consumption and Risk of Coronary Heart Disease in Women: Prospective Cohort Study," *British Medical Journal* 317 (14 November 1998), 1341–1345.

J. Sabate et al., "Effects of Walnuts on Serum Lipid Levels and Blood Pressure in Normal Men," *New England Journal of Medicine* 328 (4 March 1993), 603–607.

Daniel Zambón et al., "Substituting Walnuts for Monounsaturated Fat Improves the Serum Lipid Profile of Hypercholesterolemic Men and Women," *Annals of Internal Medicine* 132 (4 April 2000), 538–546.

Christine M. Albert et al., "Nut Consumption and Decreased Risk of Sudden Cardiac Death in the Physicians' Health Study," *Archives of Internal Medicine* 162 (24 June 2002), 1382–1387.

S. Rajaram and J. Sabate, "Nuts, Body Weight and Insulin Resistance," *British Journal of Nutrition* 96 (November 2006), S79–S86.

P. Garcia-Lorda et al., "Nut Consumption, Body Weight, and Insulin Resistance," *European Journal of Clinical Nutrition* 57 (September 2003), S8–S11.

L. Andersen et al., "Consumption of Coffee Is Associated with Reduced Risk of Death Attributed to Inflammatory and Cardiovascular Diseases in the Iowa Women's Health Study," *American Journal of Clinical Nutrition* 83 (May 2006), 1039–1046.

Eduardo Salazar-Martinez et al., "Coffee Consumption and Risk for Type 2 Diabetes Mellitus," *Annals of Internal Medicine* 140 (1 January 2004), 1–8.

Roy Walford, *Beyond the 120-Year Diet: How to Double Your Vital Years* (New York: Four Walls Eight Windows, 2000).

Roy Walford and Lisa Walford, *The Anti-Aging Plan: The Nutrient-Rich, Low-Calorie Way of Eating for a Longer Life—The Only Diet Scientifically Proven to Extend Your Healthy Years* (New York: Marlowe, 2005).

Barbara Rolls and Robert Barnett, *The Volumetrics Weight Control Plan: Feel Full on Fewer Calories* (New York: Harper Collins, 2000).

Center for Science in the Public Interest, "Fresh Mex: Not Always Healthy Mex," press release, 30 September 2003, http://www.cspinet.org/new/200309301.html.

*Nutrition Action Health Letter* 33, no. 9 (November 2006), 8.

## Chapter 6
## Mental Health: Live Better, Live Longer

R. B. Shekelle et al., "The MRFIT Behavior Pattern II: Type A Behavior and Incidence of Coronary Heart Disease," *American Journal of Epidemiology* 122 (October 1985), 559–570.

T. M. Dembroski et al., "Components of Hostility as Predictors of Sudden Death and Myocardial Infarction in the Multiple Risk Factor Intervention Trial," *Psychosomatic Medicine* 5 (September–October 1989), 514–522.

Johan Denollet et al., "Type D Personality: A Potential Risk Factor Identified," *Journal of Psychosomatic Research* 49 (October 2000), 255–266.

Johan Denollet et al., "Inadequate Response to Treatment in Coronary Heart Disease: Adverse Effects of Type D Personality and Younger Age on 5-Year Prognosis and Quality of Life," *Circulation* 102 (8 August 2000), 630–635.

Johan Denollet et al., "Personality as Independent Predictor of Long-Term Mortality in Patients with Coronary Heart Disease," *Lancet* 347 (17 February 1996), 417–421.

Thomas T. Perls, Margery Hutter Silver, with John F. Lauerman, *Living to 100: Lessons in Living to Your Maximum Potential at Any* Age (New York: Basic Books, 2000).

V. A. Barnes, F. A. Treiber, and M. H. Johnson, "Impact of Transcendental Meditation on Ambulatory Blood Pressure in African-American Adolescents," *American Journal of Hypertension* 17 (April 2004), 366–369.

S. Sivasankaran et al., "The Effect of a Six-Week Program of Yoga and Meditation on Brachial Artery Reactivity: Do Psychosocial Interventions Affect Vascular Tone?" *Clinical Cardiology* 29 (September 2006), 393–398.

Nancy Frasure-Smith et al., "Depression and 18-Month Prognosis after Myocardial Infarction," *Circulation* 91 (15 February 1995), 999–1005.

Harry Hemmingway and Michael Marmot, "Evidence Based Cardiology: Psychosocial Factors in the Aetiology and Prognosis of Coronary Heart Disease: Systematic Review of Prospective Cohort Studies," *British Medical Journal* 318 (29 May 1999), 1460–1467.

D. D. Danner, D. A. Snowdon, and W. V. Friesen, "Positive Emotions in Early Life and Longevity: Findings from the Nun Study," *Journal of Personality and Social Psychology* 80 (May 2001), 804–813.

Y. Barak, "The Immune System and Happiness," *Autoimmunity Reviews* 5 (October 2006), 523–527.

John F. Helliwell and Robert D. Putnam, "The Social Context of Well-Being," *Philosophical Transactions of the Royal Society, Series B: Biological Sciences*, 359 (29 September 2004), 1435–1446.

Lisa F. Berkman and S. Leonard Syme, "Social Networks, Host Resistance, and Mortality: A Nine-Year Follow-Up Study of Alameda County Residents," *American Journal of Epidemiology* 109 (February 1979), 186–204.

Teresa E. Seeman et al., "Social Network Ties and Mortality Among the Elderly in the Alameda County Study," *American Journal of Epidemiology* 126 (October 1987), 714–723.

Victor J. Schoenbach et al., "Social Ties and Mortality in Evans County, Georgia," *American Journal of Epidemiology* 123 (April 1986), 577–591.

David G. Myers, *The Pursuit of Happiness: Discovering the Pathway to Fulfillment, Well-Being, and Enduring Personal Joy* (New York: Harper Paperbacks, 1993).

## Chapter 7
## Tobacco: Quit Now, Here's How

U.S. Department of Health and Human Services, *Surgeon General's Report: Reducing the Health Consequences of Smoking,* 1964, http://www.cdc.gov/tobacco/sgr/sgr_1964/sgr64.htm.

P. M. Fischer et al., "Brand Logo Recognition by Children Aged 3 to 6 Years: Mickey Mouse and Old Joe the Camel," *JAMA: The Journal of the American Medical Association* 266 (11 December 1991), 3145–3148.

J. R. DiFranza et al., "RJR Nabisco's Cartoon Camel Promotes Camel Cigarettes to Children," *JAMA: The Journal of the American Medical Association* 266 (11 December 1991), 3149–3153.

K. Michael Cummings et al., "Are Smokers Adequately Informed About the Health Risks of Smoking and Medicinal Nicotine?" *Nicotine and Tobacco Research* 6 (December 2004), S333–S340.

Jyoti D. Patel, Peter B. Bach, and Mark G. Kris, "Lung Cancer in U.S. Women: A Contemporary Epidemic," *JAMA: The Journal of the American Medical Association* 291 (14 April 2004), 1763–1768.

U.S. Department of Health and Human Services, *Women and Smoking: A Report of the Surgeon General* (Washington, D.C.: Public Health Service, Office of the Surgeon General, 2001).

Hirohiko Morita et al., "Only Two-Week Smoking Cessation Improves Platelet Aggregability and Intraplatelet Redox Imbalance of Long-Term Smokers," *JACC: Journal of the American College of Cardiology* 45 (15 February 2005), 589–594.

U.S. Department of Health and Human Services, "2004 Surgeon General's Report— The Health Consequences of Smoking: Within 20 Minutes of Quitting" (Washington, D.C.: Public Health Service, Office of the Surgeon General, 2004).

U.S. Department of Health and Human Services, *The Health Benefits of Smoking Cessation: A Report of the Surgeon General* (Rockville, Md.: Public Health Service, Centers for Disease Control, 1990).

Xianglan Zhang et al., "Association of Passive Smoking by Husbands with Prevalence of Stroke Among Chinese Women Nonsmokers," *American Journal of Epidemiology* 161 (1 February 2005), 213–218.

Konrad Jamrozik, "Estimate of Deaths Attributable to Passive Smoking Among UK Adults: Database Analysis," *British Medical Journal* 330 (9 April 2005), 812–815.

Richard P. Sargent, Robert M. Shepard, and Stanton A. Glantz, "Reduced Incidence of Admissions for Myocardial Infarction Associated with Public Smoking Ban: Before and After Study," *British Medical Journal* 328 (24 April 2004), 977–980.

Richard J. Flanigan, "Recommendation for Cigarette Smoking Cessation," *The American Journal of Cardiology* 83 (1 June 1999), 1592–1593.

## Chapter 8
## Alcohol: Friend and Foe

Serge Renaud and M. deLorgeril, "Wine, Alcohol, Platelets, and the French Paradox for Coronary Heart Disease," *Lancet* 339 (20 June 1992), 1523–1526.

R. C. Ellison et al., "Lifestyle Determinants of High-Density Lipoprotein Cholesterol: The National Heart, Lung, and Blood Institute Family Heart Study," *American Heart Journal* 147 (March 2004), 529–535.

Serge Renaud and M. deLorgeril, "Wine, Alcohol, Platelets, and the French Paradox for Coronary Heart Disease," *Lancet* 339 (20 June 1992), 1523–1526.

John B. Standridge, Robert G. Zylstra, and Stephen M. Adams, "Alcohol Consumption: An Overview of Benefits and Risks," *Southern Medical Journal* 97 (July 2004), 664–672.

Joline W. J. Beulins et al., "Alcohol Consumption and Risk for Coronary Heart Disease Among Men with Hypertension," *Annals of Internal Medicine* 146 (2 January 2007), 10–19.

Ira J. Goldberg et al., "Wine and Your Heart: A Science Advisory for Healthcare Professionals from the Nutrition Committee, Council on Epidemiology and Prevention, and Council on Cardiovascular Nursing of the American Heart Association," *Circulation* 103 (23 January 2001), 472–475.

Roger Corder et al., "Endothelin-1 Synthesis Reduced by Red Wine," *Nature* 414 (20 December 2001), 863–864.

James H. Stein et al., "Purple Grape Juice Improves Endothelial Function and Reduces the Susceptibility of LDL Cholesterol to Oxidation in Patients with Coronary Artery Disease," *Circulation* 100 (7 September 1999), 1050–1055.

Joseph A. Baue et al., "Resveratrol Improves Health and Survival of Mice on a High-Calorie Diet," *Nature* 444 (16 November 2006), 337–342.

A. Ruano-Ravina, A. Figueiras, and J. M. Barros-Dios, "Type of Wine and Risk of

Lung Cancer: A Case-Control Study in Spain," *Thorax* 59 (November 2004), 981–985.

W. M. Schoonen et al., "Alcohol Consumption and Risk of Prostate Cancer in Middle-Aged Men," *International Journal of Cancer* 113 (1 January 2005), 133–140.

U.S. Centers for Disease Control and Prevention, "Quick Stats: General Information on Alcohol Use and Health," http://www.cdc.gov/alcohol/quickstats/general_info.htm.

## Chapter 9
## Medications and Supplements: What to Take

M. R. Law, N. J. Wald, and A. R. Rudnicka, "Quantifying Effect of Statins on Low-Density Lipoprotein Cholesterol, Ischaemic Heart Disease, and Stroke: Systematic Review and Meta-analysis," *British Medical Journal* 326 (28 June 2003), 1407–1408.

David D. Waters, "What the Statin Trials Have Taught Us," *The American Journal of Cardiology* 98 (1 July 2006), 129–134.

Gregory G. Schwartz et al., "Effects of Atorvastatin on Early Recurrent Ischemic Events in Acute Coronary Syndromes: The MIRACL Study—A Randomized Controlled Trial," *JAMA: The Journal of the American Medical Association* 285 (4 April 2001), 1711–1718.

G. Brown et al., "Regression of Coronary Artery Disease as a Result of Intensive Lipid-Lowering Therapy in Men with High Levels of Apolipoprotein B," *New England Journal of Medicine* 323 (8 November 1990), 1289–1298.

Gregory G. Schwartz et al., "Effects of Atorvastatin on Early Recurrent Ischemic Events in Acute Coronary Syndromes: The MIRACL Study—A Randomized Controlled Trial," *JAMA: The Journal of the American Medical Association* 285 (4 April 2001), 1711–1718.

M. Raikou et al., "Cost-Effectiveness of Primary Prevention of Cardiovascular Disease with Atorvastatin in Type 2 Diabetes: Results from the Collaborative Atorvastatin Diabetes Study (CARDS)," *Diabetologia* 50 (April 2007), 733–740.

James S. Forrester and Peter Libby, "The Inflammation Hypothesis and Its Potential Relevance to Statin Therapy," *The American Journal of Cardiology* 99 (1 March 2007), 732–738.

N. J. Wald and M. R. Law, "A Strategy to Reduce Cardiovascular Disease by More Than 80 Percent," *British Medical Journal* 326 (28 June 2003), 1419.

Oscar H. Franco et al., "The Polymeal: A More Natural, Safer, and Probably Tastier (Than the Polypill) Strategy to Reduce Cardiovascular Disease by More Than 75 Percent," *British Medical Journal* 329 (18 December 2004), 1447–1450.

B. Neal, S. MacMahon, and N. Chapman, "Effects of ACE Inhibitors, Calcium Antagonists, and Other Blood Pressure–Lowering Drugs: Results of Prospectively Designed Overviews of Randomised Trials—Blood Pressure–Lowering Treatment Trialists' Collaboration," *Lancet* 356 (9 December 2000), 1955–1964.

A. V. Chobanian et al., "Seventh Report of the Joint National Committee on Prevention, Detection, Evaluation, and Treatment of High Blood Pressure," *Hypertension* 42 (December 2003), 1206–1252.

"Final Report on the Aspirin Component of the Ongoing Physicians' Health Study: Steering Committee of the Physicians' Health Study Research Group," *New England Journal of Medicine* 321 (20 July 1989), 129–135.

Rebecca D. Jackson et al., "Calcium Plus Vitamin D Supplementation and the Risk of Fractures," *New England Journal of Medicine* 354 (16 February 2006), 669–683.

D. P. Vivekananthan et al., "Use of Antioxidant Vitamins for the Prevention of Cardiovascular Disease: Meta-analysis of Randomized Trials," *Lancet* 361 (14 June 2003), 2017–2023.

## Chapter 10
## Simple Tests: Monitor Your Health

P. Hopkins et al., "Association of Coronary Artery Calcified Plaque with Clinical Coronary Heart Disease in the National Heart, Lung, and Blood Institute's Family Heart Study," *The American Journal of Cardiology* 97 (1 June 2006), 1564–1569.

Philip Greenland and J. Michael Gaziano, "Selecting Asymptomatic Patients for Coronary Computed Tomography or Electrocardiographic Exercise Testing," *New England Journal of Medicine* 349 (31 July 2003), 465–473.

Pablo Denes et al., "Major and Minor ECG Abnormalities in Asymptomatic Women and Risk of Cardiovascular Events and Mortality," *JAMA: The Journal of the American Medical Association* 297 (7 March 2007), 978–985.

Donna L. Hoyert et al., "Deaths, Final Data for 2003," *National Vital Statistics Reports* 54, no. 13 (April 2006).

L. A. G. Ries et al., *SEER Cancer Statistics Review, 1975–2003*, National Cancer Institute, Bethesda, Md., http://seer.cancer.gov/csr/1975_2003/.

C. I. Henschke et al., "Survival of Patients with Stage I Lung Cancer Detected on CT Screening," *New England Journal of Medicine* 355 (26 October 2006), 1763–1771.

Peter B. Bach et al., "Computed Tomography Screening and Lung Cancer Outcomes," *JAMA: The Journal of the American Medical Association* 297 (7 March 2007), 953–961.

E. Rand Sutherland and Reuben M. Cherniack, "Management of Chronic Obstructive Pulmonary Disease," *New England Journal of Medicine* 350 (24 June 2004), 2689–2697.

National Osteoporosis Foundation, "Osteoporosis: Bone Density," http://www.nof.org/osteoporosis/bonemass.htm.

Christopher Nielson, Theodore Lange, and Nicholas Hadjokas, "Blood Glucose and Coronary Artery Disease in Nondiabetic Patients," *Diabetes Care* 29 (May 2006), 998–1001.

G. L. Booth et al., "Relation Between Age and Cardiovascular Disease in Men and Women with Diabetes Compared with Non-diabetic People: A Population-Based Retrospective Cohort Study," *Lancet* 368 (1 July 2006), 29–36.

## Chapter 11
## Longevity Made Simple: Putting It All Together

Goran Bjelakovic et al., "Mortality in Randomized Trials of Antioxidant Supplements for Primary and Secondary Prevention: Systematic Review and Meta-analysis," *JAMA: The Journal of the American Medical Association* 297 (28 February 2007), 842–857.

# INDEX

# ABOUT THE AUTHORS

**Richard J. Flanigan, MD**

Dr. Flanigan is an assistant clinical professor of cardiology at the University of Colorado Health Sciences Center and a private practitioner. He lectures frequently and has served as president of the Colorado Chapter of the American Heart Association. He is also co-director of the Heart and Health Prevention Center in Denver, Colorado, and a world champion rower.

**Kate Flanigan Sawyer, MD, MPH**

Dr. Flanigan Sawyer is co-director of the Heart and Health Prevention Center and a reviewing medical officer for the Department of Health and Human Services, Federal Occupational Health Division. She is also founder and CEO of Colorado Prevention Consultants, LLC.

Visit www.longevitymadesimple.com for more information on the authors.